Infection control in the built environment

DESIGN AND PLANNING

London: The Stationery Office

Published by TSO (The Stationery Office) and available from:

Online
www.tso.co.uk/bookshop

Mail, Telephone, Fax & E-mail
TSO
PO Box 29, Norwich NR3 1GN
Telephone orders/General enquiries 0870 600 5522
Fax orders 0870 600 5533
E-mail book.orders@tso.co.uk

TSO Shops
123 Kingsway, London WC2B 6PQ
020 7242 6393 Fax 020 7242 6394
68–69 Bull Street, Birmingham B4 6AD
0121 236 9696 Fax 0121 236 9699
9–21 Princess Street, Manchester M60 8AS
0161 834 7201 Fax 0161 833 0634
16 Arthur Street, Belfast BT1 4GD
028 9023 8451 Fax 028 9023 5401
18–19 High Street, Cardiff CF10 1PT
029 2039 5548 Fax 029 2038 4347
71 Lothian Road, Edinburgh EH3 9AZ
0870 606 5566 Fax 0870 606 5588

TSO Accredited Agents
(see Yellow Pages)

and through good booksellers

ISBN 0-11-322086-3

First published 2001; second edition 2002

Printed in the United Kingdom for The Stationery Office

"If the burden of healthcare-associated infection is to be reduced, it is imperative that architects, designers and builders be partners with healthcare staff and infection control teams when planning new facilities or renovating older buildings."

This guidance supersedes the Infection Control guidance published June 2001. Please disregard all previous editions, including that available on the Building Better Healthcare 2 CD-Rom 2001.

Explanation of amendments

The revised guidance does not constitute a substantial rewriting of the original guidance. The structure of the original has been preserved. A full list of all the amendments has not been included, but an outline of major changes are the following:

- Section 4 – which deals with important functional areas, activity spaces, and services to be addressed when designing and planning healthcare facilities – has been expanded upon in greater detail. In addition, a list of recommendations has been included at the end of each sub-section, summarising the salient points.

- For ease of reference, these lists of recommendations are consolidated within the Executive Summary at the beginning of the guidance.

- An infection control risk assessment tool to be used when planning construction/refurbishment of a healthcare facility has been included in the appendices. It details the measures to be taken according to scale of work and type of department.

An in-depth infection control literature review is included at the end of the main references classified according to specialty or clinical area.

Executive summary and recommendations

Research and investigation have consistently confirmed that the healthcare environment is a secondary reservoir for organisms with the potential for infecting patients. If healthcare-associated infection is to be reduced, it is imperative that infection control is "designed-in" at the planning and design stages of a healthcare-facility new-build or renovation project and that input continues up to the final build stage.

Designed-in infection control means that designers, architects, engineers, facilities managers and planners work in collaborative partnership with infection control teams to deliver facilities in which infection control needs have been planned for, anticipated and met.

This guidance discusses the various stages of a capital build project from initial concept through to post-project evaluation, and highlights the major infection control issues and risks that need to be addressed at each particular stage to achieve designed-in infection control.

The principles of this guidance can be applied to all healthcare facilities. Although the specific recommendations or processes it outlines may not necessarily be relevant to all types of healthcare facility or organisation, they may become more applicable as certain healthcare services and functions are decentralised.

The most important points raised by the document are that there is:

- a need for timely, collaborative partnership to achieve infection control goals specific to each construction project;

- a need to understand and assess the risks of infection relating to construction projects and the built environment;

- a need for all stakeholders to understand the basic principles of "designed-in" infection control;

- a need for good project management in relation to infection control considerations for all new-build and refurbishment projects;

- a need for quality control throughout the duration of the construction project;

- a need to continually monitor developments.

RECOMMENDATIONS

The following is a summary of principles underpinning, and of key considerations that would assist in achieving, designed-in infection control. The lists are grouped according to important functional areas, activity spaces and services to be addressed when designing and planning healthcare premises. These are expanded upon in Chapter 4.

Sizing/space

- Bed centres should be at least 3.6 m apart (NHS Estates' 'Ward layouts with privacy and dignity'). Bed groupings should contain the smallest possible number of beds.

- There should be sufficient single rooms to prevent patients known to be a risk for spreading infections being "housed" in open ward areas. Trusts should audit use of single rooms to determine where requirements are greatest.

- Initial planning and design in new builds needs to include numbers of beds and the appropriate space required between beds in accordance with the type of clinical intervention to be undertaken in the immediate patient environment.

- Beds in a cohort should be kept to the minimum number possible, as this will greatly assist in the prevention of cross-infection. Single rooms would appear to be the optimum solution, but other considerations such as cost and staffing levels may preclude this. Where large numbers of beds are grouped in bays, more single rooms will be needed.

- Design, accessibility and space in patient areas all contribute to ease of cleaning and maintenance.

- Spacing must take into account access to equipment around the bed and access for staff to hand-wash facilities.

- Consideration can be given to the use of permanent screens between bed spaces as an aid to prevent frequent traffic and thus the potential for micro-organism transfer.

- Healthcare facilities must provide enough sanitary facilities and showers/bathrooms to ensure easy access, convenience and independence where possible.

- Toilet facilities should be no more than 12 m from the bed area or dayroom.

Isolation rooms/single rooms/ventilation

- With an increase in antibiotic-resistant bacteria and immunocompromised in-patients, there is an increasing need for en-suite single rooms and negative or positive pressure isolation rooms. Provision of isolation/single rooms will help prevent the spread of organisms, especially those transferred by the airborne route or those easily disseminated into the immediate patient environment.

- En-suite single rooms provide greater privacy and are preferred by many patients.

- Single rooms can also be used for isolating patients with communicable diseases.

- Isolation rooms should have a hand-wash sink in the ante-room, the isolation room itself and the en-suite facility.

- Isolation requirements must be considered during the design of new hospitals or renovation of existing build.

- Rationale for isolation of infectious patients should be based on an understanding of the epidemiology of an outbreak and how organisms spread from source to other patients or staff.

- On occasions it may be necessary to prioritise the use of isolation and single rooms. In such situations consideration must be given to cohort barrier nursing patients within small 2/4 bed bays. Trusts should measure themselves against the above and seek to achieve the highest standards during their refurbishment programs.

Clinical sinks

- A minimum of one hand-wash sink in each single room is required. En-suite single rooms should have a hand-wash basin in the en-suite facility in addition to a clinical hand-wash basin in the patient's room.

- Isolation rooms should have a hand-wash sink in the ante-room, isolation room and en-suite facilities.

- Ideally, in intensive care and high dependency units (critical care areas), consideration should be given to providing one hand-wash basin at the front of each bed space (see NHS Estates' HBN 57, 'Critical care facilities').

- In acute, elderly and long-term care settings, consideration should be given to providing one sink between four patients.

- In low-dependency settings, for example mental health units and learning disability units, consideration should be given to providing one sink between six patients.

- In out-patient areas and primary care settings, a hand-wash basin must be close to where clinical procedures are carried out.

- Hand-wash sinks must be accessible and must not be situated behind curtain rails.

- All toilet facilities must have a hand-wash sink.

- The use of hand-wash sinks for purposes other than hand-washing must be discouraged.

- Wall-mounted cartridge soap/antibacterial agent dispensers and paper towels must be available at each hand-wash sink.

- Elbow-operated or non-touch mixer taps are required for all clinical hand-wash sinks.

- Hand-wash sinks must be designed for that purpose.

- Hand-wash sinks must not have a plug or overflow or be capable of taking a sink plug.

- The taps must not be aligned to run directly into the drain aperture.

- Waterproof splashbacks should be used for all sinks.

- Space must be allowed at the design stage for the placement of waste bins next to the hand-wash basin.

- Separate, appropriately-sized sinks must be installed, where required, for decontamination. Two sinks will be needed: one for washing and one for rinsing, plus a hand-wash basin.

Ancillary areas

- Ancillary areas provided as part of a ward, department, primary care facility or community home must be easily accessible, fit for the purpose, and safe, both from a health and safety and from an infection control perspective.

- The infection control issues in an ancillary area must be included along with other design features and will depend on what the ancillary area is to be used for, who will have access, and what type of activity will be carried out there.

- Ancillary areas must be easily cleaned, have facilities for hand-washing, disposal of fluid and clinical waste, if appropriate, and sufficient storage for supplies and equipment.

- Clean and dirty areas must be kept separate, and the workflow pattern and management of each area must be clearly defined.

Engineering services

- Heat emitters should be designed and installed in a manner that prevents build up of dust and contaminants.

- Heat emitters, heating and general ventilation grilles should be easily accessible for cleaning.

- Ventilation should dilute airborne contamination by removing contaminated air from the room or immediate patient vicinity and replacing it with clean air from the outside or from low-risk areas within the healthcare building.

- Lighting should be planned so that lamps can be easily cleaned, with no ledges or ridges where dust can gather.

- The use of vacuum-controlled units with overflow protection devices for mechanical suction is essential to avoid contaminating the system with aspirated body fluid.

- Contamination of the water supply can occur due to poor design of pipework, inappropriate storage or during renovation and refurbishment work. Such problems can be overcome by:

    (i)   cleaning water-storage tanks,

    (ii) maintaining a consistently high temperature in hot-water supplies or introducing a form of online disinfection (chlorine dioxide, ionisation) if lower temperature hot water is used to avoid thermostatic mixing valves and scalding (see Health & Safety Commission, 2001);

    (iii) maintaining plant regularly, minimising dead-legs;

    (iv) keeping cold water systems cold; and

    (v)   minimising water storage (NHS Estates' HTM 2027 and HTM 2040).

- *Protection of patients with special needs:* patients who have a lowered immune response are also at risk from certain organisms found in water supplies in hospital, and will need to be protected from this problem with particular attention to drinking water and washwater facilities.

- Ice for the immunocompromised should be made by putting drinking water into single-use icemakers, then into a conventional freezer.

Storage

- Patients need lockers or wardrobes for their personal possessions and clothing.

- Domestic cleaning equipment, laundry and clinical waste need to be stored in separate purpose-built areas to prevent cross-contamination.

- All healthcare premises need a storage area for large pieces of equipment such as beds, mattresses, hoists, wheelchairs and trolleys which are not currently in use.

- Sufficient and appropriate storage will not only protect equipment from contamination and dust which may potentially carry micro-organisms, but also allow free access to floors and shelves for domestic cleaning.

Finishes and floors, walls, ceilings, doors, windows, interior design, fixtures and fittings

- The quality of finishes in all areas should be of a high standard, and cost allowances in HBNs make due recognition of this need. Guidance on the selection of finishes is provided in several HTMs.

- Soft furnishings must be covered in an impervious material within all clinical and associated areas.

- Flooring should be smooth, easily cleaned and appropriately wear-resistant.

- The use of carpets is **not** advised within any clinical or associated area. Attractive vinyl flooring materials are available which can provide aesthetic appeal.

- All joints and crevices should be sealed.

- Curtains must be able to withstand washing processes at disinfection temperatures.

- Window blinds should be used with caution; the need for regular cleaning in clinical areas must be considered.

- All surfaces should be designed for easy cleaning.

- Smooth, hard, impervious surfaces should be used for walls.

- All surfaces, fittings, fixtures and furnishings should be designed for easy cleaning and durability.

Decontamination

- In order to review elements in the built environment which impact on decontamination of surgical instruments and other re-usable medical devices which are invasive by intent, it is necessary to look at the whole life-cycle of surgical instruments.

- The process assessment tools in the 'Decontamination Programme – Technical Manual' act as a useful checklist for planning areas in the built environment which are involved in purchasing, processing, maintaining, storing and using medical devices.

- Local reprocessing should be the exception rather than the norm, and facilities should therefore be designed with adequate and appropriate storage for centrally-provided sterile supplies.

Laundry and linen services

- Linen has to be disinfected during laundering and rendered free of vegetative pathogens. In this way, prevention of infection of both patients and staff is achieved.

- Large quantities of linen produced in healthcare establishments can only be dealt with effectively in large industrial washers and tumble-dryers.

- In both hospitals and the laundry, there should be separate storage areas for clean laundry and used laundry which is awaiting collection or decontamination.

- Used linen should be divided at source into three categories (used linen, heat labile linen and infectious linen) and bagged in appropriately colour-coded bags before sending to the laundry.

- There is a need to carefully segregate used linen from clean linen in commercial laundries or launderettes. The work should flow from dirty to clean areas. Consideration should be given as to whether different-coloured uniforms should be

supplied to discourage staff from moving from one area to another.

- Where launderettes are provided in hospitals for long-stay patients, the following areas should be considered:

  1. The infection control department must be involved in the planning and design of any new launderettes.

  2. The area to be used must be specifically designated as a launderette and no other activities must be carried out there, for example eating or smoking.

  3. The walls and floor must be washable and internal decoration must be to an acceptable standard.

  4. Washers and dryers of an industrial standard must be purchased (domestic washing machines have a very small rinse cycle). Washers must have a sluice and disinfection cycle and dryers must be vented to outside.

  5. The machines should be sited on a plinth so that pumps can be omitted. (These are a potential cross-infection risk.)

  6. There must be segregation of clean and dirty linen and sufficient storage facilities for both.

  7. There must be provision of a separate hand-wash basin and all necessary protective clothing such as gloves, aprons etc.

- Washing machines must incorporate temperature-recording equipment which is regularly monitored and calibrated.

- There must be appropriately-sited hand-wash basins in sufficient quantity and with easy access for staff.

- Staff changing rooms and sanitary facilities should be provided for male and female staff. There must be access to a shower room.

- Infection control teams should be included in the review and auditing of healthcare contracts.

Catering/food hygiene

- All healthcare establishments must comply with the food safety requirements in the Food Safety Act 1990 and food hygiene regulations made under this Act.

- There are many requirements when planning or upgrading a new catering facility. The Department of Health's 'Health Service Guidelines: management of food hygiene and food services in the NHS' and 'Hospital catering: delivering a quality service' both give useful guidance. Initial planning and design meetings should include the local authority environmental health inspector, key managers and the infection control team.

- When deciding on the location of the building, it is important to remember that there will be regular deliveries to the kitchen from outside suppliers. It is essential that delivery vehicles can gain easy access and catering staff are able to monitor the delivery temperature and unpack and store the food quickly. Similarly, there must be prompt distribution of food trolleys from the kitchen to the serving areas.

- A first consideration should be to establish the type of catering that will be provided; for example, the regeneration of frozen food will require different facilities from those needed for the preparation of fresh food.

- The facility must be large enough to cater for the number of meals and the type of food production.

- The layout, design and construction must be designed to ensure that high standards of cleaning and disinfection can be maintained. The finishes to walls, floors, work surfaces and equipment must be capable of withstanding regular cleaning and the impact of mechanical cleaning equipment.

- There must be separation of the processes for handling raw and cooked food and separation of "clean" and "dirty" activities (food preparation and dishwashing).

- Food preparation areas must be physically separated from the store for the cleaning equipment, and from sanitary facilities.

- There should be adequate facilities for the safe storage, at correct temperature, of raw, fresh and cooked frozen foods. It may be necessary to include cooling rooms/larders for controlled cooling before refrigeration, blast chillers for rapid cooling, thawing cabinets for controlled thawing, chilled vegetable stores, chilled service units, ice-making equipment and heat lamps over bains-marie.

- It must be possible to monitor the correct temperature of a process from equipment used (for example, that dishwashers achieve thermo-disinfection).

- An adequate number of suitably located hand-wash basins must be provided.

- Each hand-wash basin and every sink provided must have an adequate supply of hot and cold water.

- Drains must be adequate for the purpose.

- The ventilation must be sufficient to maintain a comfortable environment for the staff and prevent the premises and equipment from overheating. Artificial ventilation systems must be constructed to permit access for cleaning and maintenance. Condensation will encourage the growth of mould.

- Precautions should be taken to prevent the entry of insects, rodents and other pests into any area of food storage or preparation.

- The disposal of food waste must be separated from the food preparation area and be pest- and rodent-proof. A water supply and floor-level drainage are required to deal with spillages and for cleaning.

- Staff toilets and changing rooms with showering facilities should be provided (NHS Estates' HBN 10).

- *Ward kitchens, pantries and therapeutic kitchens:* equipment purchased must conform to the standards in the Food Safety Act and regulations under the Act. This includes the need for a separate hand-wash basin and finishes used for the floors, walls, etc. The size and design will vary according to the overall decision for food preparation in the premises. If a cook-chill system or regeneration of frozen food is to take place, the kitchen will need to be larger to house the regeneration oven and will need additional ventilation.

- The reprocessing of crockery and cutlery is achieved more effectively with a central dishwashing facility in the hospital setting.

Waste – segregation, storage and disposal

- Systems in place must be capable of protecting patients, staff, contractors and the environment from harm.

- The risk of invasive injury and contamination by blood and body fluids increases if waste is not segregated/ stored and disposed of correctly. Cost and risk are therefore the prime motivation for improvement in primary waste disposal practice and for the provision of facilities in the built environment to accomplish it.

- *Storage/disposal hold:* the storage facilities provided will vary with type of healthcare facility and method of final disposal.

- Future strategies will need to include green issues in disposal of clinical waste.

Changing facilities

- Changing facilities should be provided for staff, to encourage them to change out of their uniform in the workplace. They will also need to be able to store their personal belongings safely while on duty.

- Hand-wash basins and sanitary facilities should be included, and showers should be provided in the event of contamination by blood or body fluid.

Service lifts/pneumatic delivery systems

- It is important during a planning stage and when refurbishment work is to be undertaken to remember that hospitals have their own unique traffic patterns. These will vary according to the nature of the departments being served, relative locations of lift entrances, links to other buildings and the type of patients/staff/visitors using the areas.

- In some locations, traffic groups can be segregated to optimise on efficiency, degree of urgency and to provide some degree of privacy for patients, that is, theatre traffic, accident and emergency traffic or high dependency patients.

- The carrier for specimens should be transparent, able to be autoclaved and incorporate a leak-proof seal.

- If leaking samples are allowed to enter the tube system or station the station should be isolated and dealt with following advice from the infection control team. The disinfection procedure or cleaning will depend on the nature and level of risk imposed by the contaminant. Each incident will need to be assessed separately.

- Major policy decisions with reference to the system should be made through the infection control committee.

Design for a safe, clean environment

- Areas to consider are:

  - surfaces that facilitate easy cleaning (smooth, hard, impervious floor finishes, benches, walls and ceilings);

  - welded/sealed joints to prevent water egress;

  - sealed skirting boards;

  - low dust retention fixtures/fittings;

  - splash-backs to sinks and in-tact seals around sinks;

  - adequate storage facilities for equipment not in use;

  - bed storage/cleaning facilities;

  - storage for cleaning equipment;

  - adequate supplies of equipment and PPE;

  - colour-coded segregation of cleaning equipment;

  - communication and time to clean additional areas such as isolation rooms/bays involved in outbreaks;

  - induction and regular in-service training;

- Accommodation must be provided where cleaning equipment can be cleaned and stored. This facility should include a slop-hopper sink for disposal of potentially contaminated cleaning water. Hand-washing facilities are also required.

Construction and the role of cleaning

- A planned cleaning programme is essential when building work of any nature is planned.

- Workflow and agreed time-scales are important to prevent incidents that potentially put patients/ clients at risk.

- Frequent auditing (visual and microbiological) of the area involved will highlight any problems.

- Early involvement of the infection control team in the planning process will alleviate potential infection control risks.

Acknowledgements

NHS Estates gratefully acknowledges all contributions to this publication.

Particular thanks are due to the author:

Sue Wiseman, Infection Control Nursing Adviser, Public Health Laboratory Service, Dorset County Hospital, West Dorset NHS Trusts

NHS Estates would also like to thank the following members of the Working Group who generously donated their time to offer their expert advice and consultation on drafts:

John Barker, Manager, Sterilization & Disinfection Unit, Derriford Hospital, Derriford, Plymouth

Carole Fry, Nursing Officer Communicable Diseases, Department of Health

Dr Adam Fraise, Advisor to the Medical Devices Agency, Department of Medical Microbiology, City Hospital NHS Trust, Birmingham

Dawn Hill, Nurse Consultant Infection Control, Frenchay Hospital, North Bristol NHS Trust, Bristol

Sheila Morgan, Chair, Infection Control Nurses Association, Freeman Hospital, Newcastle upon Tyne

Sue Privett, Senior Lecturer in the Public and Community Health Department, School of Health Care, Oxford Brookes University, Oxford

Dr Robert C. Spencer, Chairman Central Sterilising Club, Bristol Public Health Laboratory, Bristol

Dr Mark H. Wilcox, Consultant & Head of Microbiology Leeds Teaching Hospitals, Reader in Medical Microbiology, University of Leeds, Leeds

Kate Woodhead, Chair, National Association of Theatre Nurses, 6 Grove Park Court, Harrogate, North Yorks

Thanks are also due to all those who commented on the draft during the consultation period:

Geoff Callan, Chair, Health Facilities Management Association (HEFMA)

Ruth Gelletlie, Chair, Public Health Medicine Environmental Group

Helen Glenister, Medical Devices Agency

Marjorie Greig, Honorary Secretary, Hospital Infection Society

Mary Henry, Consultant Nurse Epidemiologist, Scottish Centre for Infection and Environmental Health

Frances Hirst, Health & Safety Executive

Peter Hoffman, Laboratory of Hospital Infection, Central Public Health Laboratory

Howarth Litchfield Partnership, Architects, County Durham

Dee May, Infection Control Adviser, Royal College of Nursing

Dick Mayon-White, Consultant in Public Health, Oxford Health Authority

William R. Pym, Secretary, The Institute of Healthcare Engineering and Estate Management (IHEEM)

Mike Simmons, Health & Social Services Committee, National Assembly for Wales

Peter White, Principal Inspector, Drinking Water Inspectorate

Contents

Introduction

This document's principal aim is to provide guidance on the prevention of cross-infection in healthcare facilities to those responsible for the planning, design and maintenance of such facilities. It is therefore intended as a first point of reference on infection control for healthcare estates and facilities managers, architects, builders, engineers, surveyors, health planners and infection control teams working on healthcare estate new-build and refurbishment projects. It will also be useful as a guide for best practice in existing healthcare facilities.

It is not an infection control manual, nor is it intended as a comprehensive guide to the principles underpinning the global issues surrounding infection control.

ORIGINS

The idea for a generic document on infection control in relation to healthcare facilities was born out of the need to pull together information that is already available, but not always widely known, on infection control topics relating to the planning, design and maintenance of buildings for healthcare estates and facilities, and to bring this relevant information to those who need to know.

At the inception of a new-build or refurbishment project, infection control and its implications for planning and design have all too often been overlooked, leading, in some cases, to costly alterations and delays further down the line. Thus, this document will clearly define the planning process with the aim of promoting early – and continual – collaboration between all key project members.

PURPOSE

The document aims to:

- encourage timely communication between professionals involved in the planning, design and maintenance of healthcare buildings where prevention of cross-infection in healthcare premises and infection control issues impinge upon project management;

- outline the Department of Health's initiatives and policies that underpin present infection control practice related to the planning, design and maintenance of healthcare buildings for both refurbishment and new-build;

- draw together the present guidance on infection control, contained in NHS Estates documents, for healthcare estates and facilities managers, architects, builders, engineers, surveyors, health planners and infection control teams working on health estates projects;

- act as a valuable resource for refurbishment projects or new-build and as guidance for existing buildings.

The document includes references to pertinent literature and other sources, but does not provide an exhaustive literature search.

STRUCTURE

The document is structured to enable the reader to access the relevant points quickly and easily and, where only brief information has been included, highlight further useful references.

1 Background

This chapter provides an overview of Department of Health initiatives and policies that impact both on the prevention of cross-infection in healthcare premises and on healthcare estates and facilities management.

2 Infection control risk management

This chapter outlines the infection control implications for planning construction and renovation, and where risk assessment will help to mitigate environmental sources of microbes and prevention of infection through architectural design.

Controls assurance is also discussed in this chapter.

3 Understanding the planning process

The planning process is explained, and each professional's responsibility during the project in relation to infection control issues is discussed.

A project development chart of the process is included.

4 Planning and designing a healthcare facility: issues to consider

A planning guide is provided as a checklist for quick and easy access to the relevant areas of interest in the planning process. It is suggested that each area is checked against the project plans at the appropriate time in the design and planning process (see the project development chart in Chapter 3). Timing will vary from project to project, but the suggested time-scale will aid the novice involved in the planning of a healthcare building for the first time.

Appendices

Appendix 1

This includes a brief description of problem organisms, with the emphasis on routes of transmission in the built environment and methods of control or prevention.

Appendix 2

This section includes an infection control risk assessment to undertake during construction/refurbishment of a healthcare facility.

Appendix 3

This section illustrates the capital investment process for healthcare facilities and is taken from the 'Capital Investment Manual', a Department of Health publication that represents a comprehensive approach to the planning and delivery of capital schemes.

Appendix 4

This describes the four categories of equipment supplied for new building schemes.

Appendix 5

A draft pro-forma for capital planning and infection control projects is included, which can be photocopied and adapted for users' own projects.

Appendix 6

Summary of principles and approach to infection control.

Appendix 7

Glossary of terms used in the guidance.

References (and further reading)

Infection control in specialist settings – literature review

1 Background

1.1 "In today's healthcare arena, changes are occurring so rapidly and dramatically that yesterday's trends will not be tomorrow's trends, causing one to stay fluid and flexible as strategies for the future are developed."

(R Clayton McWhorter in 'Hospital and Healthcare Facility Design')

1.2 The profile of infection control in the NHS has been raised significantly in recent years. The Implementation Programme for the NHS Plan (December 2000) (Department of Health, 2000, http://www.doh.gov.uk/ nhsplanimpprogramme) makes it clear that all organisations must have effective systems in place to prevent and control healthcare-associated infection. There have also been major reports on the subject from the National Audit Office (February 2000) and the House of Commons Committee of Public Accounts (November 2000). The importance of infection control in tackling the universal problem of antimicrobial resistance has been made clear in reports on that subject from the House of Lords Select Committee on Science and Technology (March 1998 and March 2001) and the Standing Medical Advisory Committee (September 1998) (Department of Health, 1998, http://www.doh.gov.uk/ smac1.htm).

1.3 In addition to these, there have been many books and articles written on the subject – but none have issued comprehensive guidance on infection control as it relates to healthcare-facility construction and renovation projects.

1.4 Extant guidance and research on infection control issues are disseminated across a broad range of publications worldwide, making search and retrieval of material time-consuming, unwieldy and often non-productive for those seeking timely information. This book seeks to redress the balance and provide an up-to-date, "first stop" guidance for all those involved in the design and planning stages of such healthcare building projects by reviewing and collating this fragmentary wealth of knowledge on infection control and outlining its implications for the built environment. This is a crucial part of the action and strategy to tackle and reduce healthcare-associated infection.

THE BUILT ENVIRONMENT, QUALITY CARE AND IMPLICATIONS OF THE NHS PLAN

Infection control and the built environment

1.5 Owing to major technical and therapeutic advances, the control of infection in healthcare today has become an even greater challenge than ever before. In addition, microbial resistance has become a major public health threat, making infections difficult to treat and sometimes resulting in life-threatening complications or a prolonged stay in hospital.

1.6 Although they have common aims, architects, planners and trust chief executives increasingly find themselves having to come to a compromise to include every requirement when building a modern healthcare facility as there are many conflicts of interest:

- patient-centred healthcare and efficiency needs;

- finance and "humanising" the environment (for example, furnishing health premises with works of art); and

- infection control needs, space constraints and aesthetics.

1.7 The design demands of emerging technologies also conflict with the need to control and contain resistant organisms that cause cross-infection.

1.8 Furthermore, the lifespan of healthcare facilities has contracted and buildings may be reconfigured for other uses several times during their existence. This becomes more difficult or complex depending on their original design or use, for example:

- single rooms without en-suite facilities to isolation rooms;

- a six-bedded bay converted to a pacing room;

- a primary care consulting room to a minor surgery area.

1.9 Research and investigation have consistently confirmed that the healthcare environment is a secondary reservoir for organisms with the potential for infecting patients. Thus, if this burden of healthcare-associated infection is to be reduced, it is imperative that architects, designers and builders be partners with healthcare staff and infection control teams when planning new facilities or renovating older buildings.

Infection control and quality care

1.10 Good risk management awareness and practice at all levels is a critical success factor for any organisation (see Chapter 2). Risk is inherent in everything that an organisation does, for example:

- treating patients;

- managing projects;

- processing equipment;

- purchasing new medical equipment;

- managing services such as water supply and wastewater, ventilation, waste disposal and laundering;

- environmental pollution control, etc.

1.11 Clinical governance is the driving force behind the Government's strategy for improving quality in the NHS. It is defined as "a framework through which NHS organisations are accountable for continuously improving the quality of their services and safeguarding high standards of care by creating an environment in which clinical care can flourish" ('A First Class Service', Department of Health). In other words, it aims to ensure that patients receive safe care practices that are up to date and timely. Risk assessment, organisational control and clinical governance frameworks all need to be integrated to support the operation of a successful infection control policy.

Infection control and the NHS Plan

1.12 The most recent development in the Government's NHS policy – the NHS Plan, introduced in July 2000 (http://www.nhs.uk/nationalplan) – followed a wide consultation process involving patients, the public and healthcare workers, and promises far-reaching changes across the NHS. The purpose and vision of the Plan is to give the people of Britain a health service fit for the twenty-first century – a health service designed around the patient. To accomplish this it will need facilities that are cost-effective, practical and to the standards that patients expect. Many of the existing buildings, both in primary and secondary care, were built in an era when healthcare was very different from that of today; as already mentioned, future healthcare design has to incorporate the ever increasing technological advances and changing methods in medical treatment.

1.13 There are huge challenges ahead for architects, planners, hospital managers and those staff with responsibility for advising on infection control issues.

Investment has to accompany these reforms and cost containment will still play a major role in the redevelopment or upgrading of healthcare buildings.

1.14 Tomorrow's healthcare will also be consumer-driven and it is the convenience of the patient rather than that of the provider which will drive facility design. There will be an increasing emphasis on decentralising facilities for certain types of care, for example minor surgery, and these facilities will not only need to be patient-friendly but also offer a safe environment for quality care. Healthcare building design will need to facilitate such care, but be informed by evidence-based research too.

GOVERNMENT INITIATIVES AND POLICIES: THE ROLE OF INFECTION CONTROL IN HEALTHCARE TODAY

1.15 Guidance on the control of infection in hospitals has dwelt mainly on management arrangements required (see HSG(95)10: 'Hospital infection control' (Department of Health, 1995). Since this date, there have been developments in healthcare practice which have led to a decline in in-patient population and a concomitant rise in out-patient or ambulatory services. Additionally, for in-patients, length of stay has decreased but vulnerability to infection has increased.

1.16 The impact of healthcare-associated infection has, however, remained a real concern and the success of hospital infection control programmes focused on the areas of major risk and present management structures are increasingly being questioned.

Health Service Circulars (HSCs)

1.17 These are documents produced by the Department of Health setting out specific action on the part of recipients with a deadline where appropriate.

1.18 A number of HSCs issued during 1999–2000 highlighted the need to strengthen arrangements for the prevention and control of infection in hospitals and to tackle antimicrobial resistance as a major threat to public health. Those circulars also set out action required of the NHS in both areas to minimise the risk of infection for patients and staff in healthcare settings and are relevant to the issues discussed in this document.

1.19 The following HSCs particularly impact on infection control, the built environment or management of facilities.

HSC 1999/049 – Resistance to antibiotics and other antimicrobial agents

1.20 This circular followed a major House of Lords Science and Technology Select Committee report and recommendations. In its response the Government gave a commitment to taking forward a wide range of actions aimed at reducing the emergence and spread of antimicrobial resistance and its impact on treatment of infection.

1.21 The HSC sets out action for the NHS to:

- minimise morbidity and mortality due to antimicrobial-resistant infection, including hospital-acquired infection;

- contribute to the control of antimicrobial-resistant organisms, so facilitating more efficient and effective use of NHS resources.

HSC 1999/123 – Controls assurance statements 199/2000: risk management and organisational controls

1.22 This requires NHS trusts and health authorities to report on risk management and organisational controls. Eighteen controls assurance standards were listed, including one on infection control, and were based on existing statutory, mandatory and best/good practice guidance. The standards integrate the many and varied existing requirements into a common framework and for the first time infection control is included with other systems of operational management with which it has close links. Controls assurance is seen as a process designed to provide evidence that NHS bodies are doing their reasonable best to manage themselves so as to meet their objectives and protect patients, staff, the public and other stakeholders from risks of all kinds.

1.23 Risks do not always fit neatly into one category only, nor do they always restrict themselves to one group of people; thus, controls assurance appears to be the first guidance which has tried to integrate risk management into the whole organisation. This encourages communication between infection control personnel, estates departments, health and safety departments, audit committees and human resources departments so creating an environment in which quality and high standards of care for patients can flourish. This impacts on issues discussed in later chapters.

HSC 2000/002 – The Management and Control of Hospital Infection

1.24 This circular sets out a programme of action for the NHS to:

- strengthen prevention and control of infection in hospital;

- secure appropriate healthcare services for patients with infection;

- improve surveillance of hospital infection;

- monitor and optimise antimicrobial prescribing.

1.25 It complements HSC 1999/049 'Resistance to Antibiotics and other Antimicrobial Agents' and the controls assurance framework.

1.26 Among its eight objectives are securing a safe, clinical environment and appropriate provision of isolation facilities. This can only be achieved by the infection control team's involvement in service specifications and the planning process for healthcare buildings or renovation. This guidance document will help to inform infection control teams in this planning process.

HSC 2000/032 – Decontamination of Medical Devices

1.27 This circular identifies the short- and medium-term actions required to ensure decontamination of medical devices is carried out effectively and sets out the information required to gather a robust picture of decontamination provision across the NHS.

The Socio-economic Burden of Hospital-acquired Infection

1.28 The aim of this study (Plowman et al, 2000, http://www.doh.gov.uk/haicosts.htm), commissioned by the Department of Health, was to assess the burden of hospital-acquired infection in terms of the costs to the public sector, patients, informal carers and society as a whole.

1.29 The study looked at the costs to secondary and primary healthcare as well as community care services and evaluated the specific costs for different types of hospital-acquired infection. Its aim was to identify those patients at greatest risk of incurring highest costs and to predict the effects of hospital-acquired infection on these cost categories.

1.30 It provides background information on the extent of the problem of hospital-acquired infection and detailed aims, objectives and methods used. It also provides key sample characteristics for the various groups of patients studied, i.e. in-patients and post-discharge patient episodes. Cost analysis is given for the hospital and primary care sector and for patient personal expenditure on drugs, dressings, travel, etc.

1.31 Analysis is undertaken on patient and informal carers' days lost to productive activity. The impact hospital-acquired infection has on health status is also analysed along with in-patient mortality and the value of years of life lost.

1.32 Estimates are made of the gross benefits that might result if the incidence of hospital-acquired infection observed in the study could be reduced by 10%. The study presents recommendations arising from the research.

1.33 The report helps to highlight the substantial problems of hospital-acquired infection and the gross benefits of prevention as represented by the value of resources available for other use. On the basis of experience at the one study hospital, the researchers estimate that the annual burden of hospital-acquired infections to the NHS is around £1 billion per annum. The report concludes that further research is needed to establish the net benefits of alternative infection control practices and programmes.

1.34 Prevention of infection through attention to the built environment and facilities management is just one area that can help reduce the potential for the spread of organisms that contribute to this problem.

Report by the Comptroller and Auditor General: The Management and Control of Hospital-acquired Infection in Acute NHS Trusts in England – February 2000

1.35 This report (National Audit Office, 2000, http://www.nao.gov.uk/publications/nao_reports/9900230es.pdf) refers to published research which found that, at any given time, around 9% of patients have an infection acquired after their admission to hospital (equivalent to at least 100,000 infections per year), causing them to suffer discomfort, prolonged or permanent disability and even death.

1.36 The cost of treating these infections is discussed in the previous report 'The Socio-economic Burden of Hospital-acquired Infection'. The Comptroller and Auditor General estimates, from information provided by infection control teams, that across all NHS trusts, infection rates could be reduced by 15% by better application of existing knowledge and realistic infection control policies.

1.37 The report investigates the strategic management of hospital-acquired infection, what is known about the extent and cost of HAI and how well hospital-acquired infections are controlled through prevention, detection and containment measures in acute NHS hospital trusts in England. The main focus of the investigation is the work of the NHS trust's infection control team and a key part of the methodology was a census of these trusts.

1.38 One of its many conclusions was that infection control has implications for the whole hospital, and the advice of the infection control team is important in ensuring that the risk of infection is minimised. One of its recommendations to NHS trusts is that infection control teams should be consulted when equipment is purchased, alterations are planned or new hospitals are to be built and contracts let or renewed. Infection control teams, together with the Consultant in Communicable Disease Control (CCDC), are also more involved in infection control in the community and this

trend will increase with the increase in the amount of day-care surgery, out-patient invasive procedures and early patient discharge from hospitals.

UK Antimicrobial Resistance Strategy and Action Plan (June 2000)

1.39 This Department of Health document (http://www.doh.gov.uk/arbstrat.htm) sets out the Government's comprehensive three-year strategy and the key actions required to tackle the problem of antimicrobial resistance. The strategy recognises the need for action across a wide range of interests and by many organisations and individuals.

1.40 The action areas discussed include:

- general – commitment from all players: local, national and international;

- surveillance;

- prudent antimicrobial use in humans, animals and other spheres;

- infection control;

- information technology;

- research.

1.41 Infection control and the built environment is one of the areas that will need to be managed as part of the bigger picture to strengthen infection control practices and processes in hospitals and the community.

Risks associated with hospital-acquired infections

1.42 'The Commons Public Accounts Committee's Forty-second Report: The Management and Control of Hospital-acquired Infection in Acute NHS Trusts in England (23 November 2000)' has raised public awareness of hospital-acquired infections. The report argues that infection control procedures need to be urgently improved. The report states that there needs to be a change in philosophy such that infection control is everybody's business, not just the specialists.

1.43 Consideration of design, planning, facility layout, and finishes to surfaces, floors, walls and fittings, ventilation, shelving, bed layout should all be addressed so that some risks can be eliminated or at least significantly minimised. A list of the relevant HBNs and HTMs covering these areas is given in the References.

NHS Plan – Implementation Programme December 2000

1.44 The Implementation Programme (http://www.doh.gov.uk/nhsplanimpprogramme) states that it is a core requirement that all relevant organisations should ensure they have effective systems in place, including decontamination, to prevent and control communicable diseases – especially healthcare-associated infection – to minimise the risk to patients and others. Organisations should also take action to control and reduce antimicrobial resistance.

National evidence-based guidelines for preventing healthcare-associated infections – January 2001

1.45 Department of Health-commissioned, evidence-based guidelines for the prevention and control of healthcare-associated infection (HAI) were published as a supplement to the *Journal of Hospital Infection* and have three components:

1. Standard principles for preventing HAI.

2. Prevention of infection associated with short-term indwelling urethral catheters.

3. Prevention of infection associated with central venous catheters.

1.46 The guidelines can be found at: http://www.doh.gov.uk/hai/

RESEARCH

1.47 Evidence based on double-blind placebo controlled trials or studies is rare in infection control. Studies which look at infection control, the built environment and facilities management are even rarer!

1.48 Common questions related to the environment and planning or renovation of a healthcare building are difficult to answer if an evidence base is to be used. If the only way of judging the effectiveness of advice is based on strong evidence type I and II used by the Bandolier system, then this chapter would be very short indeed. Nevertheless, if resources are to be allocated effectively, infection control teams in partnership with architects, designers and managers need to produce clear evidence about these resources.

1.49 The research referred to throughout this guidance, in the context of infection control and the built environment, relates to type IV or V strength of evidence. It also relates to new directions observed in hospital and healthcare design today and reasonable inference about what does or does not aid patient-centred care and prevention of cross-infection in these areas.

1.50 Where there is no available research tried and tested, basic infection control principles have been applied.

2 Infection control risk management

2.1 Risk management involves three stages:

1. identifying risk;

2. assessing risk;

3. managing the identified risks by elimination or by using controls to reduce the risk.

Identifying risk

2.2 The time taken to plan or refurbish a healthcare facility can vary from a relatively short period in the case of urgent renovation to as long as three or four years for a major capital build project. It is therefore important that infection control teams are notified of capital bids or contracts to architects at the earliest possible time. The microbiologist and infection control team need to be involved in the first planning meetings. Most meetings thereafter will require some input from them.

2.3 To avoid mistakes and pitfalls, infection control teams must consider the real issues:

- How will the product, equipment, room or clinic be used?

- What possible solutions are available?

- What are the budgetary limitations?

- What infection control principles or external regulations apply?

- What does the evidence suggest in relation to the specific context?

- What are the laws governing the project?

- What are the standards and guidelines from architectural and engineering bodies, government departments and accrediting agencies?

- Which product or design best balances the infection control requirements with employee and patient safety and satisfaction, and cost constraints? (Carter and Barr, 1997).

Common pitfalls

2.4 Common pitfalls arise from a number of pressures, for example, the pressure to choose the cheapest products or design. As many authors have argued, the best products or designs may be more expensive initially but in the long term they will probably realise cost benefits as they may prevent outbreaks, or they may last longer and require less maintenance and be more durable.

Common errors

2.5 Common errors in design and construction [adapted from by Carter and Barr (1997)] due to inept or non-existent risk management include:

- Air intakes placed too close to exhausts or other mistakes in the placement of air intakes.

- Incorrect number of air exchanges.

- Air-handling system functions only during the week or on particular days of the week.

- Airvents not reopened after construction is finished.

- No negative air-pressure rooms built in a large, new inpatient building.

- Carpet placed where vinyl should be used.

- Wet-vacuum system in the operating suite pulls water up one floor into a holding tank rather than down one floor.

- Aerators on taps (also avoid swan-neck outlets where possible).

- Sinks located in inaccessible places.

- Patient rooms or treatment rooms do not have sinks in which healthcare workers and visitors can wash their hands.

- Doors too narrow to allow beds and equipment to be moved in an out of room

- Inadequate space to allow safe use of medical devices and equipment.

2.6 Carter and Barr reported these errors during construction projects they encountered in their practice of infection control, and they recommend that infection control personnel inspect the construction site frequently to make sure the workers are following the recommendations.

Assessing risk

2.7 Outbreaks of infection have been related to the design, plan, layout, function and/or finish of the built environment (Cotterill et al, 1996; Kumari et al, 1998). Thus, risk assessment is a fundamental imperative in the planning and design stages of a healthcare facility. Yet it is often overlooked or compromised throughout the lifecycle of the project. Disseminating good specialist knowledge and involving infection control teams throughout all phases of construction and renovation projects will reduce risks. Failure to assess infection control risk properly can lead to expensive redesign later and expose the patient and healthcare worker to infection control hazards.

Managing the risk

2.8 Infection control teams need to help non-clinical professionals to understand the main principles of how infection is spread in the context of the built environment. These principles should inform the design and planning stages of health service facilities projects. When evaluating the spread of infection and its control, three aspects should be considered:

1. source;

2. mode of transmission; and

3. susceptible recipient.

Source

2.9 Building professionals must be convinced about the risks associated with construction projects, and that the environment can be a reservoir for potentially infective agents. The source is the person, animal, object or substance from which an infectious agent is transmitted to a host. The immediate hospital environment can be a potential reservoir of micro-organisms and source of infection or contamination Therefore, designers and planners need to consider eliminating potential sources of infection by practising good design, for example:

- storage facilities (see "Storage" in chapter 4);

- choice of materials, avoiding unnecessary surfaces that may become reservoirs for infectious agents (see "Finishes" in chapter 4); and

- ensuring materials and surfaces can be cleaned and maintained.

2.10 It has been reported (Rampling et al, 2001) that antibiotic-resistant bacteria, such as methicillin-resistant *Staphylococcus aureus* (MRSA), may survive and persist in the environment leading to recurrent outbreaks (see the table of common infective agents associated with construction in Appendix 1).

2.11 Attention to prevention of airborne infection by the use of ventilation in specialist areas and correct engineering and mechanical services contribute greatly to reducing potential reservoirs of infection in the built environment.

2.12 Elimination of other environmental sources of infection, for example pests, litter, insects, birds, small mammals and waste, should be considered at the outset of a project and reviewed throughout. Common pests include rats, mice, ants, cockroaches, pigeons and flies. All carry micro-organisms on their bodies and in their droppings. Hospital hygiene is dependent on controlling pests.

Mode of transmission

2.13 A basic understanding of modes of transmission of infection assists in promoting joint responsibility for infection control. Micro-organisms can be transmitted in three main ways:

- **direct** transmission involving direct transfer of micro-organisms to the skin or mucous membranes by direct contact;

- **indirect** transmission involving an intermediate stage between the source of infection and the individual, for example infected food, water or vector-borne transmission by insects;

- **airborne** transmission involving inhaling aerosols containing micro-organisms, for example legionnaires' disease or tuberculosis.

2.14 Environmental dispersal of micro-organisms during construction, resulting in healthcare-associated infections, should also be emphasised to non-medical members of the project teams.

2.15 There is a need to assess the infection risks during construction and how construction activity itself may be a mechanism for infection; for example, environmental airborne contaminants and infectious agents are closely related to water and moisture conditions and figure prominently in construction activity. (See Appendix 2 for an infection control risk assessment to be carried out during construction/refurbishment of a healthcare facility.)

Susceptible recipient

2.16 Preventing transmission of infectious agents to vulnerable patient populations, healthcare workers and visitors is an important component of infection control programmes.

2.17 Outbreaks affecting immunocompromised patients have been reported, and construction professionals need to understand the concept of the at-risk patient. Some groups of patients are especially susceptible to certain infectious agents to which they may be exposed in the hospital construction environment (see Appendix 1).

CONTROLS ASSURANCE

2.18 Controls assurance is a process designed to provide evidence that NHS organisations are doing their "reasonable best" to manage themselves so as to meet their objectives and protect patients, staff, the public, and other stakeholders against risks of all kinds. The Department of Health's Health Service Circular 1999/123 'Controls Assurance Statements 1999/2000: Risk Management and Organisational Controls' requires trusts and health authorities to report on risk management and organisational controls.

2.19 Controls assurance was introduced to encourage communication between the:

- infection control team,
- estates department,
- health and safety department,
- audit committees,
- human resources departments, and particularly,
- planning and design departments,

so creating an environment in which quality and high standards of patient care can flourish. Certain standards form part of the controls assurance framework; they relate to an area of potentially significant risk for an NHS organisation and are subject to ongoing monitoring and review. The current standards are on the latest issue of the Controls Assurance CD-ROM (sent separately to all relevant NHS organisations, and also available from the NHS Response Line on 0541 555 455) and are downloadable from the controls assurance website: (http://www.doh.gov.uk/riskman.htm). (See Criterion 4 of the Department of Health's Infection Control Controls Assurance Standard, which is particularly relevant to the planning process.)

CONCLUSION

2.20 The integration of infection control risk management and construction is in its infancy. It represents a significant change in the management of healthcare facilities design and planning that will take time to develop to a level at which the greatest benefits can be achieved. Just as important then is the need to carry out research in the area of risk management, infection control and the built environment to produce sound irrefutable evidence on which to base further risk management strategies. The guidance outlined in chapter 4 aims to demonstrate, in general terms, the areas where basic infection control principles and risk management, if applied, will promote prevention of cross-infection in the built environment.

IMPORTANT

- Always consult the infection control team at an early stage:

    - Whenever refitting or refurbishment is planned

    - Whenever major capital bids are planned.

- Do not wait until patients are ready to move in.

- Do not wait until fixtures, fittings and furnishings have been purchased.

- Do not let cost or space consideration override reason!

- Most advice will be common sense but not always popular financially.

3 Understanding the planning process

STRATEGIC PLANNING AND THE ROLE OF
INFECTION CONTROL

3.1 In England, there are no regulations prescribing that infection control personnel must participate in strategic planning for construction. In the USA, the current authority for construction design for federal and healthcare providers is the 1996–1997 edition of the 'Guidelines for Design and Construction of Hospital and Healthcare Facilities', published by the American Institute of Architects/Academy of Architecture for Health (1996) with assistance from the US Department of Health and Human Services. The latest version strongly supports infection control input at early planning and design stages.

3.2 For infection control teams to effectively participate in the planning process for both renovation and new-build, it is necessary for them to understand the process from its inception to completion.

Project roles and responsibilities

3.3 A comprehensive approach to planning needs to include consultation with inclusion of the appropriate specialists from its inception through to post-project evaluation.

Key project roles

3.4 The project organisation should comprise:

1. trust internal organisation (see "Project Organisation", 'Capital Investment Manual', Department of Health):[1]

   - trust board

     (should monitor cost and progress of all capital investment projects at regular meetings. If problems are identified, it needs to be satisfied that appropriate steps are being taken);

   - chief executive officer

     (given the project-specific role, title, and responsibility of project owner);

- project board

  (comprising senior staff within the trust who have an interest in the project and whose activities will be affected by the project, for example staff from clinical areas such as infection control);

- project director

  (responsible for project management);

- professional adviser

  (experienced in construction and design, especially of healthcare facilities);

- user panel

  (representatives of each of the relevant service departments, in each case authorised to define their department's needs and to review and agree how those needs are to be met).

2. External resources:

   - project manager;

   - other consultants.

HEALTH AND SAFETY LEGISLATION AND
INFECTION CONTROL

3.5 It is important to remember that many of the recommendations in this guidance, while evidenced-based, may also be required by health and safety law in respect of controlling the risk of infection to staff and patients. This needs to be taken into account during the process of planning, designing and maintaining healthcare premises as this will clearly influence the final outcome. The following outlines some of the key features of relevant legislation which impinge on the control of infection.

Health and Safety at Work etc Act 1974

3.6 The duties of employers under the Health and Safety at Work etc Act 1974, that is, to protect the health, safety and welfare of employees, extend to patients and others who may be affected by work – this includes control of infection measures.

---

1 As this document is being produced, the 'Capital Investment Manual' is being rewritten to guide the huge investment plan for new healthcare build agreed in the NHS Plan

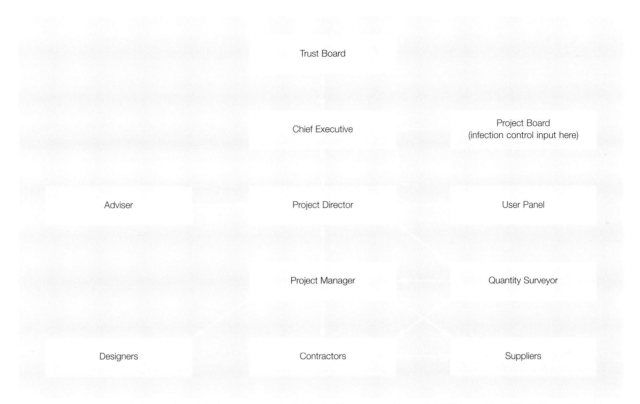

Trust Board

Chief Executive

Project Board
(infection control input here)

Adviser

Project Director

User Panel

Project Manager

Quantity Surveyor

Designers

Contractors

Suppliers

Management structure (adapted from "Project organisation", 'Capital Investment Manual', NHS Executive, 1994) (Reproduced by kind permission of the Department of Health)

3.7 Anyone involved in the supply of equipment, plant or machinery for use at work has to make sure that, as far as is reasonably practicable, it is safe and does not cause any risk to health when used at work. For example:

- equipment should be made of materials that can easily be disinfected and which do not support microbial growth;

- plant or equipment which needs regular cleaning should be easy to access and/or easy to dismantle.

The Construction, Design and Management (CDM) Regulations 1994 (as amended)

3.8 These regulations require that health and safety is taken into account and managed throughout all stages of a project, from conception, design and planning through to site work and subsequent maintenance and repair of the structure. These regulations apply to most common building, civil engineering and engineering construction work (including demolition, dismantling and refurbishment).

3.9 The NHS body has client responsibilities under these regulations; it has to pass relevant information reasonably available to them about health and safety matters which relate to the project to those who are responsible for planning the project.

3.10 Designers also have duties under CDM:

- they should ensure that when they design for construction they assess the foreseeable health and safety risks during construction as well as the eventual maintenance and cleaning of the structure in the balance with other design considerations such as aesthetics and cost. This can be achieved by applying the normal hierarchy of risk control;

- they should identify all the hazards inherent in carrying out the construction work and, where possible, alter the design to avoid them. If the hazards cannot be removed by changing the design, then the risks will need to be controlled and the designer should provide information about the remaining risks.

The Control of Substances Hazardous to Health Regulations 1999

3.11 COSHH provides a framework for controlling the risks from most hazardous substances, including biological agents (that is, the risk of infection).

3.12 COSHH requires that employers assess the risk from all infectious agents to both their employees and others who may be affected by their work, for example patients. The assessment needs to be suitable and sufficient and must cover the steps that need to be taken to meet the requirements of the rest of the regulations. This means that the assessment should also review the use of control strategies, the maintenance and use of control measures such as air handling systems and air filtration, health surveillance requirements and – perhaps most importantly – information, instruction and training for employees. The employer is required to protect employees as far as is reasonably practicable and commensurate to the risk.

3.13 There are a number of general measures in COSHH relating to the control of exposure to biological agents which must be applied in the light of the results of the assessment. Some may impinge directly on the process of designing, planning and maintaining healthcare premises and these are highlighted in bold. The other procedural/management control measures must also be applied if employers are to fully meet their duties under COSHH:

- keeping as low as practicable the number of employees exposed or likely to be exposed to biological agents;

- **designing work processes and engineering control measures so as to prevent or minimise the release of biological agents into the place of work;**

- displaying a biohazard sign and other relevant warning signs;

- drawing up plans to deal with accidents involving biological agents;

- specifying appropriate decontamination and disinfection procedures;

- **instituting means for the safe collection, storage and disposal of contaminated waste, including the use of secure and identifiable containers, after suitable treatment where appropriate;**

- **making arrangements for the safe handling and transport of biological agents, or materials that may contain such agents, within the workplace;**

- specifying procedures for taking, handling and processing samples that may contain biological agents;

- **providing collective protection measures and, where exposure cannot be adequately controlled by other means, individual protection measures including, in particular, the supply of appropriate protective clothing or other special clothing;**

- where appropriate, making available effective vaccines for those employees who are not already immune to the biological agent to which they are exposed or liable to be exposed;

- **instituting hygiene measures compatible with the aim of preventing or reducing the accidental**

transfer or release of a biological agent from the workplace, including, in particular –

- **the provision of appropriate and adequate washing and toilet facilities** and

- the prohibition of eating, drinking, smoking and application of cosmetics in working areas where there is a risk of contamination by biological agents.

3.14 "Appropriate" in relation to clothing and hygiene measures means appropriate for the risks involved and the conditions at the workplace where exposure to the risk may occur.

THE PLANNING PROCESS

3.15 This section explains the planning process which comprises the following stages:

1. the concept/feasibility study,

2. sketch plans,

3. the preparation of a business case to support the viability of the project,

4. project funding,

5. the design stage,

6. project monitoring,

7. commissioning the facility

8. post-project evaluation.

3.16 Its aim is to prompt those with overall responsibility for managing capital schemes or private finance initiatives (PFI/PPP) to include infection control advice at the right time in order to prevent costly mistakes.

3.17 These points will now be expanded upon in more detail.

Concept/feasibility study

3.18 The planning process starts with the identification of a "need" by the users. The development of this need will involve feasibility studies to enable a design brief or output specification to be developed. The infection control team should review operational policies and procedures at this stage and there may be some 1:200 scale designs to give a broad overview of the scheme. The infection control team needs to consider:

- what effect additional beds or departments will make to policies such as waste disposal, linen, catering, domestic services etc;

- the effect of extra theatres on disinfection services, workflow etc;

- additional specialist areas in that they will probably require extra infection control and laboratory input as well as specialist advice that may not be available in-house;

- bed space and size of departments etc, plus engineering facility needs such as ultra-clean ventilation, showers versus baths etc;

- hot and cold water usage and impact on existing heating capacity and water treatment regimen.

Sketch plans

3.19 The remaining 1:200 scale designs will be available at this stage and the infection control team needs to give a broad view of infection control issues such as:

- rooms missing;

- wards without ancillary areas.

3.20 Additional considerations at this point will include:

- storage;

- ancillary areas;

- single rooms;

- isolation rooms;

- changing facilities;

- lifts;

- pneumatic delivery systems.

The business case

Outline business case

3.21 The preparation of a business case is the process that supports NHS trust submissions for funding of new capital projects (an overview of the capital investment process is given in Appendix 3). A business case must convincingly demonstrate that the project is economically sound, is financially viable (affordable to the trust and purchasers) and will be well managed. In addition, a business case for any investment should show that it will benefit patients.

3.22 The involvement and support of a wide range of managers and staff may be vital to the success of the business case, both to determine the requirement and scope of the investment and also to participate in subsequent stages of planning. It is important therefore at this stage to identify and involve key people who have a direct interest in the end product, and this will include members of the infection control team along with other leading clinicians, nursing managers and departmental heads. Specifically at this stage, infection control teams need to:

- establish the goals of infection control (what infection control risks are especially important for each specific context?);

- agree the agenda for infection control design and planning;

- communicate infection control imperatives throughout the course of the project (but especially at the initial stages);

- monitor the progress of the building/refurbishment project in relation to compliance with infection control specifications;

- determine available resources that can be used and recognise the cost benefits of not cutting corners on infection control issues.

3.23 Normally the input from the team should be managed by the project director, but for larger and more complex schemes a project manager, reporting to the project director, may be appointed to conduct the detailed work and manage the business case team.

Issues to be addressed by the infection control team

3.24 Issues frequently addressed will include costs and space constraints which will impact on areas pertinent to infection control teams, such as:

- storage and equipment cleaning areas;

- air-handling units;

- hand-washing facilities;

- furnishing and fittings;

- appropriate finishes;

- isolation rooms;

- specific products with infection control implications and applicable regulations.

Detail planning/design

3.25 It is at this stage, when the outline business case is presented, that the 1:50 scale designs will be available. There will probably be two stages to the consultation process:

1. Early on in this period the infection control team will need to review location of rooms for correct workflow/infection control practice, i.e. wards, theatres, patient passage through out-patients or primary care facilities, etc.

2. Later there will be a need to discuss the finer details such as where fixtures and fittings are located, what type of flooring, cupboards or storage systems are to be used, and ventilation in theatres, etc.

RISK MANAGEMENT (Chapter 2)

PLANNING PROCESS (Chapter 3)

Time period

- Concept
- Feasibility study — 1 — 1 in 200 (some preliminary designs)
- Sketch plans — 2 — 1 in 200: draft activity data sheets (equipment lists – usually wish-lists)
- Outline business case
- Detail planning/design — 3, 4 — 1 in 50: fixtures & fittings (fixed items in Group 1)
- Full business case
- Tender
- Contract
- Construction — 5
- Commission/Equipping — 6, 7 — Trust input to equipment budget
- Evaluation — 8

ISSUES
(paragraph numbers refer to relevant subsections in Chapter 4)

Issues to consider:
- Space (paragraphs 4.4–4.20)
- Decontamination (paragraphs 4.249–4.265)
- Specialist areas
- Engineering services (paragraphs 4.117–4.190)

Issues to consider:
- Storage (linen, waste, patient equipment, domestic equipment) (paragraphs 4.269; 4.276–4.304; 4.191–4.203)
- Ancillary areas (paragraphs 4.96–4.116)
- Changing facilities (paragraphs 4.305–4.312)
- Lifts (paragraphs 4.313–4.324)

Issues to consider:
- Ventilation (paragraphs 4.55–4.56; 4.129–4.140)
- Heating/lighting (paragraphs 4.119–4.128; 4.162–4.165)
- Water systems (paragraphs 4.141–4.161)
- Waste water and sanitation (paragraphs 4.174–4.187)
- Medical gas vacuum systems (paragraphs 4.188–4.190)

Issues to consider:
- Equipment
- Space (paragraphs 4.4–4.20)
- Specialist equipment

- Check for any changes made to original agreements/plans

STAGES OF INFECTION CONTROL INPUT

1. **Concept/feasibility study** – infection control team should review operational policies and procedures, for example 1:200 scale plans

- Adding beds to ward areas may mean extra sluice, single/isolation rooms or hand-washing facilities

- Adding extra theatres will need a review of decontamination facilities for instruments

- Additional specialist areas will need extra infection control input

2. **Sketch plans:** at this stage, the infection control team need to give a broad view of infection control issues. For example:

- Rooms missing

- Wards without ancillary areas such as disposal rooms or dirty utility

3. **Detail planning/design** (1:50 scale designs) (early period)

- There is a need to discuss locations of rooms for correct workflows/infection control practice, i.e. wards, theatres.

4. **Detail planning/design** (1:50 scale designs) (later period)

- Need to discuss finer details: location and type of fixtures and fittings, for example hand-wash basins/types of basins; airflows in theatres, flooring.

5. **Construction.** Infection control team will need input here, if new build is attached to existing healthcare building only, to prevent risks to patients.

6. **Equipment.** Decisions on equipment should be made as an ongoing process, but it is at this stage that it will be seen that previous equipment wish-lists may not fit the rooms/departments or are now outdated. It is important that infection control teams have input during this period (especially if it is a PFI/PPP build).

7. **Commission/equipping.** Infection control teams must have input during this stage if costly mistakes are not to be made.

8. **Evaluation.** This is an important stage in which lessons learnt can be highlighted for future projects.

STEPS IN THE BUSINESS CASE PROCESS

(Shaded boxes include examples of issues related to infection control that might need to be considered)

1. Set the strategic context:
    - Where are we now?
    - Where do we want to be?
    - Is it affordable?
    - In-patient/day cases
    - Single room issues
    - Controls assurance

2. Define objectives and benefit criteria:
    - Antibiotic resistance
    - Controls assurance
    - Cost benefits of preventing healthcare-associated infection

3. Generate options.

4. Measure the benefits.

5. Identify/quantify costs.

6. Assess sensitivity to risk.

7. Identify the preferred option.

8. Present the outline business case.

9. Develop the preferred option: full business case.

3.26 The team will also need to think about the infection control issues around:

1. workflow;

2. hand-wash basins and taps: types, numbers and location;

3. fixtures/fittings/flooring/furniture;

4. wastewater and sewage/body fluid disposal;

5. ventilation;

6. heating and lighting;

7. water systems;

8. suction/medical gases;

9. storage systems;

10. ward kitchens/pantry;

11. medical devices and equipment.

3.27 Point 3 in the business case process ("Generate options") should highlight the variables that drive the facility's requirements with regard to infection control. This is not always an easy task in the initial stages of a project. Table 1 gives a range of initial ideas.

Funding the project: using private finance

The private finance initiative (PFI)/public-private partnership (PPP)

3.28 The arrangements made with regard to use of privately raised capital encourage the NHS to exploit the strengths of the private sector. There are essentially two broad criteria against which all schemes are assessed: "value for money" and "assumption of risk". Trusts today are expected to explore the private finance alternative whenever a capital investment scheme is being considered. The goals of PFI/PPP are to:

- achieve objectives and deliver services more effectively;

- use public money more efficiently;

- respond positively to private-sector ideas;

- increase competition.

3.29 There are advantages for both the NHS and the private sector and these are discussed more fully in the 'Public-Private Partnerships in the National Health Service: The Private Finance Initiative' published by the Department of Health.

Key factors in PFI/PPP

3.30 The contract between the NHS purchaser and the private sector supplier is critical and it is important that the service representatives/key stakeholders and particularly in this instance the infection control team are clear about the options available and the evidence to back up any decisions they advise on. The infection control team will need to make sure that certain criteria are embedded into the contract in such a way that important decisions on design or build do not go ahead without being "signed off" by them. The team will need:

- access to all relevant and up-to-date plans and information on operational policies;

- access to any meetings deemed relevant to them or timely minutes from those meetings that they cannot attend;

- access to sites and departments as building work progresses, for example environmental rounds with checklists based on project objectives;

- regular communication between both internal project manager and the PFI/PPP team;

- involvement in decision making for any category of equipment the PFI/PPP team will purchase;

- involvement in any contracts for support services such as catering, cleaning, linen, HSDU etc that the PFI/PPP team may be providing;

- access to certain high risk areas for any microbiological testing deemed necessary, for example theatres, isolation rooms, pharmacy and HSDU clean rooms.

Design stage

3.31 It is at the design stage that infection control teams will need to follow up any input they have had in the initial brief. Sketch plans should be available to them to explain how the brief fulfils their requirements at the 1:200 and 1:50 scale design stages of the project. Suggestions for improvement in operability are encouraged at this stage. (For an approximate time-scale, see the project development chart on page 16.)

3.32 Consideration should also be given to the impact on local and existing facilities, for example ventilation and water supplies.

3.33 At this stage a legionellosis risk assessment should be carried out to ensure that any work being undertaken will not increase the risk of *Legionella* spp. in that or any local area [COSHH (1999); Health & Safety Commission (2001)].

TABLE 1 INFECTION CONTROL ISSUES TO CONSIDER IN THE CAPITAL PLANNING PROCESS (NOTE: THIS IS NOT AN EXHAUSTIVE LIST)

Accommodation areas/ internal environment/ general services	Examples
Accommodation areas	
Bed areas: • Single-bed rooms • 4-bedded bays versus 6-bedded bays	En-suite facilities • Doors on bays • En-suite facilities
Dirty utility/clean utility	Standardization of rooms Space
Workflow/layout	Standardize versus different needs of specialties
Bed planning	Elective Emergency
Linen services and facilities	Internal launderette versus commercial laundry
Catering/kitchen areas	Furnishing, fixtures and fittings plus workflow crucial for HACCP. Cook-chill versus commercial versus in-house systems
ITU/HDU	Single rooms versus 4/6/ bed bays
Handwash basins	1 to 2 versus 1 to 4 versus 1 to 6 Complete picture: sinks, taps, soap, gloves, aprons Easily accessible for staff use
Staff change areas/storage of uniforms	Type of uniform provided will dictate, i.e. "greens" versus classic
Sterilizing/disinfecting/cleaning facilities (HSDU/CSSD/TSSU)	Operational policy dictated by choice of in-house SSD or commercial facility
Equipment	Beds/mattresses Purchase versus hire Scopes/instruments Cleaning/disinfection requirement Patient-specific Enough equipment available
Priority areas: • Critical care • UCV theatres • Renal units • Hydrotherapy • Oncology • Mortuaries • Neurology • SCBUs and maternity • Paediatrics	Every specialist area will have different requirements and infection control issues so cannot be planned as standard departments
Internal environment	
Ventilation	Single rooms, bays, theatres, pacing rooms, treatment rooms, internal sanitary areas Negative- and positive-pressure isolation rooms
Heating/ventilation	Dust-free options, i.e. hidden heat panels versus radiators
Lighting	Quality as well as quantity is important The use of sealed units
Furnishings and fittings and artwork	Walls/floors/ceilings – hygiene versus aesthetics
Water	Potable Softened Water coolers/fountains
General services	
Disposal of waste	Cost versus new concepts/in-house versus commercial Storage
Communications	IT systems (timely information on pathology, etc., operational policies, infection control policies, procedures and training)
Emergency plans	Water storage if water cut off/heating /medical gases and vacuum/suction, emergency generator, ventilation, etc.
Other	
New services and expertise needed	Renal satellite units SSDs Near patient testing Hydrotherapy Pneumatic tube system Pharmacy/clean air room

Design and structure issues

3.34 These include:

- Is the facility designed to support infection control practice?

- Design, number and type of isolation rooms (i.e. airborne infection isolation or protective environments).

- Heating, ventilation, and air-conditioning systems including recommended ventilation and filtration charts.

- Mechanical/engineering/chemical systems involving water supply and plumbing.

- Number, type and placement of hand-hygiene fixtures, clinical sinks and taps, dispensers for hand-washing soap plus alcohol hand-rub, paper towels, and lotion.

- Space for waste, including sharps disposal units.

- Accommodation for personal protection equipment.

- Surfaces: ceiling tiles, walls, counters, floor covering and furnishings.

- Utility rooms: soiled, clean, holding, workrooms.

- Storage of movable and modular equipment.

- Management of waste, including clinical and biological waste.

- Linen (clean)/laundry (used)

(adapted from Bartley (2000))

3.35 Equipment schedules for groups 2 and 3 (see Appendix 4) based on room data sheets/layouts are prepared at this stage and may consist of "wish-lists" as well as equipment that is genuinely needed (it is important to remember that equipment will not be removed from lists at this stage. This will mean that at the commissioning/equipping stage many items/pieces of equipment may not fit into the finished design or are out of date before they are used). Items available for transfer should also be identified which will allow schedules for new equipment to be prepared and costed. This is an important area for input by the infection control team if costly mistakes are not to be made. (For examples of equipment groups, see Appendix 4.)

3.36 The purchase of equipment groups 2 to 4 will not normally take place until the operational commissioning period (see "Commissioning the healthcare facility/equipping" section). However, it is important during the construction and equipment supply stage that there is involvement by the infection control

team in discussion of group 2 equipment, which may have significant design implications. This will ensure that this equipment is compatible with infection control needs and also that proper inspection and testing can be agreed.

3.37 Technical commissioning of the building, services and equipment should include any areas that require inspection and testing to demonstrate compliance with infection control standards, i.e. theatres, hydrotherapy pools, isolation rooms and clean rooms in pharmacy and HSDUs.

Tender/contract

3.38 At this stage of the project, there will be little or no involvement for the infection control team.

3.39 The tender documents sent to potential companies should include any statements the trust may have about infection control that may affect the contractor's employees and the infection control requirements for the project (for example building dust controls, *Legionella* spp. control, provision of toilet and shower facilities).

Monitoring the project

Construction (new build)

3.40 If the project is a new-build, monitoring will not normally be required by the infection control team until the healthcare premises are at a stage when site visits can be arranged. It is at this point that the team should visit the site as often as possible to familiarise themselves with the layout of the various departments. This will enable them to detect any differences or problems seen.

Construction (new-build attached to existing site or refurbishment)

3.41 Infection control specialists agree that involvement of infection control teams in refurbishment projects is important not only for ensuring that "designed-in" infection control is achieved, but also for assessing the potential risks to patients in existing buildings from dust, dirt and pathogens.

3.42 Measures that may limit the spread of dust, dirt and pathogens during construction/demolition include the following: [1]

- clean and vacuum areas under construction and the surrounding areas frequently;

- place adhesive floor strips outside the door to the construction area to trap dust;

---

1 See also Hoffman et al (1999, S205–6). They provide a list of escalating control measures to reduce the incidence of fungal infection in susceptible patients during building work.

TABLE 2 DAILY CONSTRUCTION SURVEY (CARTER AND BARR 1997)

Barriers

• Construction signs posted for the area	Yes/No
• Doors properly closed and sealed	Yes/No
• Floor area clean, no dust tracked	Yes/No

Air handling

• All windows closed behind barrier	Yes/No
• Negative air at barrier entrance	Yes/No
• Negative air machine running	Yes/No

Project area

• Debris removed in covered container daily	Yes/No
• Trash in appropriate container	Yes/No
• Routine clearing done on job site	Yes/No

Traffic control

• Restricted to construction workers and necessary staff only	Yes/No
• All doors and exits free of debris	Yes/No

Dress code

• Appropriate for the area (e.g. OR, CSD)	Yes/No
• Required to enter	Yes/No
• Required to leave	Yes/No

- seal windows, doors and roof-space to control dust;

- wet-mop the area just outside the door to the construction area daily or more often if necessary;

- use a high-efficiency particulate air (HEPA) filtered vacuum to clean areas daily or more often if necessary;

- shampoo carpets when the construction project is completed;

- transport debris in containers with tightly fitting lids, or cover debris with a wet sheet;

- remove debris as it is created; do not let it accumulate. Use dust extraction equipment where feasible;

- remove debris through a window when construction occurs above the first floor;

- do not haul debris through patient-care areas;

- remove debris through an exit restricted to the construction crew;

- designate an entrance, a lift and a hallway that the construction workers must use and that are not used by patients, visitors or healthcare workers;

- commission hotel services with regard to cleaning during construction projects (adapted from Carter and Barr, 1997).

3.43 There is a need to ensure that infection control teams document advice given on building developments and that this advice is followed and recorded. A suggested pro-forma is shown in Appendix 5. Similarly, Carter and Barr (1997) advise that a daily checklist is maintained during the progress of the construction project (see Table 2). [2]

Surveillance and monitoring during renovation or construction work

3.44 Routine bacteriological sampling of floors, walls, surfaces and air is rarely indicated (Ayliffe et al, 2000) but there have been several documented outbreaks due to construction work. In 1995 there was widespread contamination of water with *Legionella pneumophila* during a period of major construction resulting in two fatal cases of healthcare-associated legionellosis (Mermel et al, 1995). Multiple outbreaks of healthcare-associated aspergillosis have also been described including one specifically attributed to hospital renovation (Flynn et al, 1993). Mermel et al (1995) suggest that heightened surveillance and preventive measures may be warranted during periods of excavation on hospital grounds or when water supplies are otherwise shut down and later repressurised.

3.45 NHS Estates (Wearmouth, 1999) advises:

Where vulnerable patients may be placed at risk, it is important that an appropriate risk assessment be carried out with the trust microbiologist/infection control officer [doctor] at an early stage in advance of

---

2 See also the Construction (Design and Management) Regulations 1994 http://www.hmso.gov.uk/si/si1994/ Uksi_19943140_en_1.htm

any demolition works or disturbance/alterations to the building fabric/ventilation systems.

3.46 Since the airborne spores of *Aspergillus* spp. can travel significant distances, this will apply generally to all works in the immediate vicinity or within the boundary of the hospital site. It is strongly advised that any recommendations by the microbiologist/infection control doctor should be incorporated into the building or engineering works so as to minimise risk.

3.47 Surveillance and monitoring during renovation or construction work may prove difficult; environmental assessment to detect *Aspergillus* spp. and to confirm epidemiological investigations may not be within the remit of all infection control teams. However, implementation of adequate infection control measures during construction are, and have been proven to be, an effective means of protecting highly susceptible or high risk patients from environmental contaminants (Thio et al, 2000).

Commissioning/equipping the healthcare facility

3.48 Upon completion of construction, the facility must be brought into use; the complexity of the task involved means that a commissioning manager and team will be needed. Senior managers, specialist teams and users should be fully involved in the process. The commissioning entails:

1. confirming operational procedures;

2. establishing baseline and future staffing profiles;

3. establishing baseline and future revenue budgets;

4. establishing equipment requirements;

5. identifying policy issues for referral to the commissioning team or the construction project team;

6. identifying staff training needs;

7. establishing the occupation programme for that user function for incorporating into the overall masterplan.

3.49 By understanding the commissioning process, infection control teams can ensure that they are included in any working groups in which their speciality will have an impact or in which requirements to modify services may have repercussions on other aspects of the prevention of infection.

3.50 The infection control team may also need to be involved in processes for:

1. transfer of facilities;

2. phased or staged occupation;

3. decorating;

4. strategy for equipping;

5. selection of equipment;

6. storage and subsequent cleaning/disinfection of any furniture or equipment;

7. commissioning hotel services for cleaning;

8. site visits;

9. artwork;

10. furnishing and fittings;

11. interior finishes and fixtures;

12. post-handover period;

13. decommissioning of redundant facilities;

14. period of handover to operational management.

Post-project evaluation

3.51 The purpose of the post-project evaluation is to improve project appraisal, design, management and implementation. It is a learning process and should not be seen as a means of allocating blame. There are three stages:

1. project appraisal;

2. monitoring and evaluation of project;

3. review of project operations. It is at the third stage when it is useful for the infection control team to be included in the evaluation teams that are reviewing project objectives. The outcomes (activity and its consequences) of the project will not be amenable to evaluation until the facility has been in use for some time.

3.52 It is important that the project is evaluated in terms of its original objectives, not in light of any new legislation or development. Performance indicators may be used if these can be measured retrospectively. Measurable objectives may include:

1. bed turnover;

2. re-admission rates;

3. incidence of day surgery;

4. activity data;

5. infection rates;

6. patient satisfaction surveys etc;

7. process measures – air sampling audit and water sampling audit.

IMPORTANT
DON'T ASSUME ANYTHING – COMMUNICATE

4 Planning and designing a healthcare facility: issues to consider

4.1 Infection control teams are often not involved in the planning process until key decisions have been made. Changes to design or equipment may then result in costly adjustments, additions or replacements.

4.2 The recommendations in this section should be applied to the planning, design and maintenance of all healthcare buildings. They offer a planning checklist that can be used throughout the design and planning process. Not all items will need to be included in every project, but using the checklist will ensure areas with infection control implications are not missed. Timing will vary from project to project but a suggested time-scale is included in Chapter 3 to help those involved in planning for the first time.

PLANNING GUIDE – AREAS WHERE INFECTION CONTROL INTERVENTIONS OR ADHERENCE TO RECOMMENDATIONS MAY HELP TO PREVENT CROSS-INFECTION

- sizing/space;

- isolation rooms/single rooms;

- clinical sinks – design for clean hands;

- ancillary areas;

- engineering and mechanical services;

- storage;

- finishes – floors, walls, ceiling, doors, windows, interior design, fixtures and fittings;

- decontamination: cleaning, disinfection and sterilization;

- laundry and linen services;

- catering/food hygiene;

- waste – segregation, storage and disposal;

- changing facilities;

- service lifts/pneumatic-air tube delivery systems;

- design for a clean, safe environment;

- construction and the role of cleaning.

4.3 This guidance can be used by anyone involved in planning. Further details can be provided by local infection control teams.

Note

For the purposes of this document, the following terminology is used:

1. **Single room** – this is a room with space for one patient and usually contains as a minimum: a bed; locker/wardrobe; and clinical hand-wash basin plus a small cupboard with worktop.

   [Clinicians use the term "side room" interchangeably with "single room", but for clarity in this document we use the term "single room".]

2. **En-suite single room** – as above but with any combination of en-suite facility, that is, shower, shower and toilet, bath and toilet or just toilet etc.

3. **Isolation room** – as in (1) and (2) but with either negative pressure ventilation for infectious patients (source isolation) or positive pressure for immunocompromised patients (protective isolation). May or may not have a lobby or en-suite facility.

4. **Bay** is any room that contains more than one bed (i.e. two-bedded bay; three-bedded bay; four-bedded bay; six-bedded bay, etc.) which may or may not have en-suite facilities.

4.4 Mode of transmission of infection (see Chapter 2) should be taken into account when bed space and size of facility is discussed. It includes direct transmission, indirect transmission via fomites (for example articles such as door handles and clothing and hospital instruments, kidney dishes, etc.) and airborne transmission. The route of spread of infection is a basic concept in cross-infection, and spacing has direct implications for the prevention of infection.

4.5 The principle should be to maintain sufficient space for activities to take place and to avoid transmission of organisms either by air or by contact with blood or body fluid or equipment. The exact space needed will vary according to numbers and activity of staff, type of patient, and environmental factors such as ventilation and humidity.

4.6 This section discusses the evidence on which recommendations to prevent overcrowding and the subsequent problems of cross-infection are based.

4.7 The areas discussed are:

1. patient groups;

2. transmission of micro-organisms:

   • avoiding cross-infection;

   • the environment and its role in cross-infection;

   • shared equipment;

   • movement of patients;

3. management issues:

   • clinical pressures;

   • inappropriate bed management;

   • shortage of single rooms.

Patient groups

4.8 Floor/bed space is influenced by the type of healthcare facility and the type of patient care. There are three distinct patient groups:

• patients requiring **acute** care, which includes trauma, multi-organ failure, medical emergencies, planned major surgery and other life-threatening emergencies plus obstetric and neonatal care;

• patients with **chronic** conditions or sub-acute conditions, which include elderly care and rehabilitation services;

• patients requiring **ambulatory** care, which includes diagnostic services, day surgery, minor injuries and attendance at primary care facilities and walk-in centres.

4.9 The first two patient groups will require in-patient care. The volume of care and the degree of intervention, diagnostic equipment and movement of staff around the patient dictates the bed space needed. (Guidance can be found in the appropriate Health Building Notes: see pages 67–68.)

4.10 Guidelines published on the design and layout of high-risk areas such as intensive care units emphasise the importance of adequate isolation rooms and also sufficient space around each bed (O'Connell and Humphreys, 2000; NHS Estates' HBN 57: 'Critical care facilities').

Transmission of organisms

Avoiding cross-infection by direct contact or airborne routes

4.11 With the increasing problems of cross-infection, there is a need to maintain sufficient space for activities to take place and avoid the risks associated with transmission of organisms from patient to patient either by the airborne route or by contact with blood, body fluid or equipment.

4.12 Direct contact and the role of the environment is discussed in relation to routes of transmission in the guidance by the Advisory Committee on Dangerous Pathogens (1995). Airborne transmission is more fully discussed in Donaldson and Donaldson (2000) and Keyworth (2000).

The environment and its role in cross-infection

4.13 Bacteria vary in their ability to survive in the environment. This ability to survive in the environment (particularly in dust found on equipment and around bed spaces) has implications for overcrowding and space management in treatment areas (Hirai, 1991; Smith et al, 1996; Lacey et al, 1986; Duckworth and Jordens, 1990; Webster et al, 1998).

4.14 The role of the environment and environmental decontamination has been the subject of many studies (Mallison and Hayley, 1981; Talon, 1999; Collins, 1988; Dennis et al, 1982). Recent studies have increasingly implicated the environment in outbreaks of cross-infection (Smith et al, 1998; Rampling et al, 2001).

4.15 Gardner and Peel (1991) and McCulloch (2000) provide a good introduction to infection control in the environment. They emphasise how the immediate hospital environment is a potential reservoir of micro-organisms and source of infection or contamination.

Shared equipment

4.16 Equipment has been implicated in the spread of infection. The long-term survival of bacteria in dry conditions has serious implications for patients with equipment used on or around them. The more confined the work area, the greater is the risk of equipment being shared between patients with the potential for further cross-infection (Barnett et al, 1999; Lambert et al, 2000; Bernard et al, 1999; Stacey et al, 1998).

Movement of patients

4.17 Moving patients between wards or departments increases the risk of cross-infection not only to the patients being moved but also to the patients with whom they come into contact. Surveillance of infection also becomes difficult.

Management issues

Clinical pressures

4.18 There is increasing pressure to reduce waiting times for both emergency admissions in accident and emergency departments and those on the waiting-list for out-patient, minor treatment, day-surgery and in-patient accommodation. This has put pressure on already overcrowded areas, which in turn increases the risks of cross-infection.

- An investigation of *Serratia marcescens* outbreak in a paediatric cardiac intensive care unit suggested that understaffing and overcrowding might have been underlying risk factors (Archibald et al, 1997).

- Haley and Bregman (1982) demonstrated that staphylococcal outbreaks periodically resulted when serious understaffing made frequent hand-washing between infants in an overcrowded neonatal nursery difficult.

- Dan (1980) linked bacteraemia to overcrowding and decreased hand-washing.

- The effect of increased bed numbers on MRSA transmission in an acute medical ward was demonstrated by Kibbler et al (1998).

- Sawyer et al (1988) [see also Chadwick et al (2000)] highlighted an outbreak of small round structured virus (SRVS) in a hospital emergency department due to overcrowding.

Inappropriate bed management

4.19 Trusts need to have a bed management system that not only helps to find the most appropriate bed for a patient (not mixing clean surgical patients with infected patients) but also helps to prevent cross-infection by tracking use of single rooms for potentially infected patients.

Shortage of single rooms

4.20 Insufficient single rooms will lead to patients with infections being "housed" in open ward areas. Green et al (1998) demonstrated in outbreaks of small round structured virus (SRSV) that cohorting infected patients [i.e. placing patients infected with the same micro-organism (but with no other infection) in a discrete clinical area where they are cared for by staff who are restricted to these patients] helps to prevent the spread of infection to other clinical areas (see "Cohort barrier nursing" in "Isolation facilities" section).

Recommendations

- Bed centres should be at least 3.6 m apart (NHS Estates' 'Ward layouts with privacy and dignity'). Bed groupings should contain the smallest possible number of beds.

- There should be sufficient single rooms to prevent patients known to be a risk for spreading infections being "housed" in open ward areas (see next section on "Isolation facilities"). Trusts should audit use of single rooms to determine where requirements are greatest.

- Initial planning and design in new builds needs to include numbers of beds and the appropriate space required between beds in accordance with the type of clinical intervention to be undertaken in the immediate patient environment.

- Beds in a cohort should be kept to the minimum number possible, as this will greatly assist in the prevention of cross-infection (Green et al, 1998). Single rooms would appear to be the optimum solution but other considerations such as cost and staffing levels may preclude this. Where large numbers of beds are grouped in bays, more single rooms will be needed.

- Design, accessibility and space in patient areas all contribute to ease of cleaning and maintenance.

- Spacing must take into account access to equipment around the bed and access for staff to hand-wash facilities.

- Consideration can be given to the use of permanent screens between bed spaces as an aid to prevent frequent traffic and thus the potential for micro-organism transfer.

- Healthcare facilities must provide enough sanitary facilities and showers/bathrooms to ensure easy access, convenience and independence where possible.

- Toilet facilities should be no more than 12 m from the bed area or dayroom.

ISOLATION ROOMS/SINGLE ROOMS

4.21 The areas discussed in this section include:

- the role of isolation/single rooms in preventing cross-infection;

- quantity;

- design:

  - hand-wash facilities;

  - sanitary facilities;

  - storage of personal protective equipment;

  - size and layout;

  - visibility/location;

  - furnishings and fixtures;

  - finishes;

  - floors;

  - walls;

  - ceilings;

  - doors;

  - windows;

  - engineering requirements;

- the cost of ignoring the advice.

The role of isolation rooms/single rooms in preventing cross-infection

4.22 The primary aim of infection control is to prevent the spread of infection between patients, visitors and staff by control or containment of potentially pathogenic organisms.

4.23 Many of these organisms can be controlled by basic infection control practices such as hand hygiene and environmental hygiene, but certain organisms can only effectively be contained by isolating the source patient.

4.24 Negative pressure isolation rooms (see definition of isolation and single rooms on page 23) are essential for infections transmitted by the airborne route: it has been reported that isolation of infected patients prevents cross-infection in outbreaks of tuberculosis (Louther et al, 1997). For other infections, a patient can be accommodated in a single room. This also provides a reminder to staff that hands should be washed – staff are less likely to go from patient to patient without washing their hands if there is this designed-in physical barrier as a reminder.

4.25 In high-risk areas where complex surgery or procedures are performed, engineering controls may need to be used. Isolation rooms are included in this group of high-risk areas. Hannan et al (2000) stress that if isolation rooms are to be used effectively, early clinical recognition is important so that patients can be isolated promptly.

Cohort barrier nursing

4.26 When an index case of infection is followed by several secondary cases, it may be necessary to cohort barrier nurse a group of patients in a bay if insufficient single rooms are available. This can be more easily achieved where wards are divided into small bays (two or four beds per bay) which can be isolated further by closure of doors at the entrance/exit and which also have en-suite facilities.

4.27 When infection control guidelines are adhered to, research has demonstrated that cohort barrier nursing can successfully control and contain infection in hospital (Cartmill et al, 1994; Zafar et al, 1998; Green et al, 1998; Karanfil et al, 1992; CDC, 1995, 1997).

Quantity

4.28 Experience has shown that many hospitals find the present allocation of isolation/single rooms inadequate to deal with the increasing numbers of infected and immunocompromised patients (Langley et al, 1994; Wiggam and Hayward, 2000). Teaching hospitals, where the prevalence of tuberculosis and MRSA is high, may need a higher than average proportion of single rooms.

4.29 Hospitals with 10% of their bed contingent as single rooms often find that this number is inadequate to cope with every infectious patient. Where this is the case, risk assessment is used to inform decisions regarding which patients to nurse in single rooms.

Negative pressure isolation rooms

4.30 As a useful method for calculating the quantity of negative pressure rooms allocated for patients with MDRTB, the former Oxford Regional Health Authority came up with the following formula of:

> providing **one** isolation room for every **100** cases of tuberculosis per year.

4.31 This is based on 1% of tuberculosis cases being due to MDRTB, and that a patient might spend up to three months in hospital before becoming smear-negative. As cases may occur in clusters, one needs to have more capacity than the straight incidence and length of stay might suggest.

4.32 This calculation has worked for the former Oxford region with a population of 2.2 million and 268 cases of tuberculosis a year: three negative pressure isolation rooms in the infectious disease unit have been enough to meet their needs.

Design

4.33 There is currently no definitive guidance on size, ventilation or the equipping of isolation rooms. NHS Estates' HBNs for relevant departments such as wards, theatres and other specialist areas and NHS Estates' HTM 2025 give advice on natural ventilation, general extract ventilation and ventilation for specialist areas.

Negative pressure isolation rooms

4.34 Annex D of the guidance produced by the Interdepartmental Working Group on Tuberculosis (1998, pp. 83–85) (http://www.doh.gov.uk/tbguide.htm) outlines features of a negative pressure isolation room used for multi-drug-resistant tuberculosis (MDRTB).

4.35 Further recommendations on design criteria for negative pressure isolation rooms are outlined in the "Guidelines for preventing the transmission of *Mycobacterium tuberculosis* in healthcare facilities" (CDC, 1994) (http://wonder.cdc.gov/wonder/prevguid/m0035909/m0035909.asp).

Hand-wash facilities

4.36 Hand hygiene and the use of PPE are key to preventing the spread of infection. Sufficient hand-wash basins must be supplied in an isolation room (and attached lobby) and single room. This is in addition to the basin provided for patient wash facilities.

4.37 Elbow taps for clinical hand-wash basins are preferred and the touch-free control of water flow will further aid the control of infection.

Sanitary facilities

4.38 Personal hygiene contributes to the prevention of cross-infection and is improved if patients have their own bath or shower, WC and hand-wash basin. Single rooms should therefore be provided with en-suite sanitary facilities. An en-suite single room should also be able to accommodate a hoist for lifting patients.

Storage of personal protective equipment (PPE)

4.39 Storage of, and ready access to, clean PPE is important to encourage its use plus appropriate clinical waste bins for its disposal once worn.

4.40 Gloves and aprons should be sited outside single rooms as organisms are spread by activity within the room and by people entering and leaving. This has the potential to contaminate such protective equipment with organisms which have the ability to survive for long periods (Neely and Maley, 2000).

Size and layout

4.41 Additional facilities may be required for the care and treatment of patients in isolation room/single rooms, especially if the isolation is likely to last for some time:

- the storage of supplies retained in the room;

- personal clothing and possessions;

- essential domestic cleaning equipment held in en-suite sanitary facilities.

4.42 Where possible, the opportunity should be taken to slightly widen the room so that the bed can be placed parallel to the external wall, thereby allowing the patient to enjoy a view of the outside. An intercommunication system, while not essential, is desirable as this allows the patient verbal contact without compromising their isolation.

Visibility/location

4.43 If patients are to stay in an isolation/single room or bay, it is important that they are able to see staff from their beds. Staff should also be able to see the patient in case of an emergency. This reduces the psychological problems of isolation. The sense of containment can also be reduced by providing outside views using windows with low sills.

Furnishing and fixtures

4.44 In isolation/single rooms/small bays where infectious patients are nursed, it is important that there be enough space to be able to clean furnishings and fixtures easily.

Finishes

4.45 Ledges, recesses and tight angles where dust particles can be trapped should be avoided to allow ease of cleaning. It should be ensured that surfaces will not be physically affected by detergents and disinfectants and that they will dry quickly.

Floors

4.46 Washable floors rather than carpets are advisable in isolation/single rooms as carpets may prolong the survival of certain organisms. (See "Carpets" section, paragraphs 4.214–4.219.)

Walls

4.47 Wall finishes should be impermeable and easily wiped over if necessary.

Ceilings

4.48 These should have homogeneous plastered surface with flush-mounted recessed lights, ventilation grilles and other ceiling fixtures. Removable ceiling tiles in a grid layout are not advised for isolation rooms.

Doors

4.49 The corridor door to the room should be one-and-half leaf and contain a large vision panel. A means of obscuring the vision panel should be included within the door.

4.50 Doors should have smooth handles which can be easily cleaned, will not be physically affected by detergents and disinfectants and will dry quickly (see NHS Estates' HTM 58).

Windows

4.51 These will need to be lockable when the specialist ventilation is turned on. Curtains to provide privacy should be controlled within the room.

Lobbies

4.52 Lobbies to isolation rooms **are not** necessary if the door to the room can be kept closed and space is provided outside the room to house protective equipment and stores.

4.53 Lobbies **are** required for isolation rooms that provide simultaneous source (negative pressure) and protective (positive pressure) isolation.

4.54 Isolation rooms used for patients with multi-drug-resistant tuberculosis (MDRTB) **must have** a lobby.

Engineering requirements for isolation rooms

4.55 *Ventilation* – provision of mechanical ventilation systems is important in controlling the required direction of air movement between isolation rooms and the adjacent corridor:

- for negative pressure isolation rooms, there should be a readily visible monitor independent of the air supply/extract system. This is best achieved by monitoring the pressure differential between the patient room and corridor or lobby. This differential should preferably be monitored continuously, i.e. an electrical monitor linked to an alarm at the nurse's station should the pressure drop below a pre-set limit. The alarm should have a built-in delay of a few seconds so that it does not activate every time the door is opened;

- for negative pressure isolation rooms, there should be an interlock system such that supply ventilation is cut off if the extract ventilation fails. There should be a clear indication to users that the ventilation has failed;

- for isolation rooms with both negative and positive pressure ventilation, the mechanism for switching from one to the other should have a lock. It should

be noted that this option of having isolation rooms with switchable ventilation is not generally recommended (except in ITUs), as infections have been transmitted through patients being cared for in a positive pressure room when they should have been in a negative pressure room. Proper training for staff on how to use the mechanism should be provided.

4.56 With regard to the en-suite sanitary facility, the extract ventilation should be as standard.

4.57 *Heating* – general space/heating requirements will be met by the same method as for "standard" single rooms. Care should be taken in selection of the heater emitter, as it needs to be easily cleaned and should not have inaccessible corners (see "Heat emitters", paragraphs 4.120–4.124).

4.58 *Lighting* – to reduce dust contamination and ease cleaning, luminaires should be recessed, dust-excluding and fully accessible from below.

4.59 *Planned maintenance and monitoring* – maintenance and monitoring programmes must be established for ventilated rooms to ensure the design criteria are maintained and met at all times. Although it is impossible to give specific maintenance frequencies, each unit must be included in a planned preventative maintenance that includes pressure/air flow monitoring equipment.

The cost of ignoring the advice

4.60 Patients with a hospital-acquired infection on average remain in hospital 2.5 times longer than an uninfected patient and incur hospital costs that are almost three times greater. Not all HAI is preventable but if success is to be achieved in prevention and subsequent reduction of HAI, facilities will need to be made available and investment will need to be made in smaller bays and isolation/single rooms. This in turn will improve the clinical outcome for patients and ensure that hospitals are equipped to deal with the problems of infection.

Recommendations

- With an increase in antibiotic-resistant bacteria and immunocompromised in-patients, there is an increasing need for en-suite single rooms and negative or positive pressure isolation rooms. Provision of isolation/single rooms will help prevent the spread of organisms, especially those transferred by the airborne route or those easily disseminated into the immediate patient environment.

- En-suite single rooms provide greater privacy and are preferred by many patients.

- Single rooms can also be used for isolating patients with communicable diseases.

- Isolation rooms should have a hand-wash sink in the ante-room, the isolation room itself and the en-suite facility.

- Isolation requirements must be considered during the design of new hospitals or renovation of existing build.

- Rationale for isolation of infectious patients should be based on an understanding of the epidemiology of an outbreak and how organisms spread from source to other patients or staff.

- On occasions it may be necessary to prioritise the use of isolation and single rooms. In such situations consideration must be given to cohort barrier nursing patients within small 2/4 bed bays. Trusts should measure themselves against the above and seek to achieve the highest standards during their refurbishment programs.

CLINICAL SINKS

4.61 Hand hygiene is the single most important factor in the prevention of healthcare-associated infection (Ayliffe et al, 2000).

4.62 It is known that hand hygiene causes a significant reduction in the carriage of potential pathogens on the hands and can result in reduction of patient morbidity and mortality from hospital-acquired infection (Pittet et al, 2000).

4.63 Compliance with hand hygiene guidelines is often poor and a contributory factor is the absence of conveniently placed sinks. Good departmental design, with sufficient hand-wash basins appropriately placed can increase compliance.

4.64 Thus, the importance of facilities to encourage hand hygiene should be high on the list of priorities when designing and planning new healthcare premises or refurbishment of existing premises is being undertaken.

4.65 This section discusses:

- design;

- sink provision;

- water/taps;

- soap/disinfection dispensers;

- hand drying;

- sinks and slop-hoppers.

Design

4.66 Sinks in clinical areas must be suitable for that purpose (not of a domestic design). Hotel-style sinks are not appropriate (HTM 64).

4.67 The dimensions of a clinical sink must be large enough to contain splashes and therefore enable the correct hand-wash technique to be performed (Bartley, 2000).

4.68 The sides of the sink should be curved to prevent splashing.

4.69 Hand-wash sinks should be sealed to the wall or placed sufficiently far from the wall to allow effective cleaning of all surfaces.

4.70 Waterproofed sink splash-backs should be included to prevent wall damage and allow ease of cleaning (Ayliffe et al, 1993, 1999).

4.71 Clinical sinks should not have a plug or a recess capable of taking a plug (NHS Estates' HBN 4 and HTM 64). A plug is an unnecessary source of infection (especially *Pseudomonas* spp.) and can discourage staff from washing their hands under running water, particularly if mixer taps are not available.

4.72 Overflows are difficult to clean and become contaminated very quickly, serving as reservoirs of bacteria. They should therefore be avoided (NHS Estates' HBN 4 and HTM 64).

Sink provision

4.73 Hand hygiene facilities must be readily available in all clinical areas. There must be sufficient sinks to encourage and assist staff to readily conform to hand hygiene protocols (Boyce et al, 2000; Feather et al, 2000; Carter and Barr, 1997; Dancer, 1999; Department of Health, 2000; Harris et al, 2000; Larson and Killien, 1982; Pittet, 2000).

4.74 Inconveniently located hand-wash facilities are one of the main reasons that healthcare staff do not comply with hand hygiene protocols (Larson and Killien, 1982; Pittet, 2000). There is a need to review the numbers and placement of sinks, as well as their dimensions (Kesavan et al, 1998; Bartley, 2000).

4.75 Guidelines for the appropriate numbers of sinks in clinical areas have been identified (NHS Estates' HBN 4). This guidance suggests a minimum of one sink per single room and small ward areas and one sink per six beds in a large multi-occupied room. However, to encourage good practice and give reasonable access, it is recommended that there should be:

- ideally, in **intensive care and high dependency units (critical care areas)**, one hand-wash basin at the front of each bed space (see NHS Estates' HBN 57: 'Critical care facilities' and also "Hand-wash facilities" in the "Isolation facilities" section, paragraphs 4.36–4.37);

- one sink between four patients in **acute, elderly and long-term care** settings; and

- one sink between six patients in **low-dependency** settings, for example mental health units and learning disability units.

4.76 In **primary care** and **out-patient** settings, where clinical procedures or examination of patients/clients is undertaken, then a sink must be close to the procedure.

4.77 NHS Estates' HTM 64 also gives details of hand hygiene facilities for other areas such as kitchens and patient wash areas.

Water/taps

4.78 Health and safety regulations [The Workplace (Health, Safety and Welfare) Regulations, 1992] require that both hot and cold running water should be available in areas where employees are expected to wash their hands.

4.79 Hands should always be washed under running water; mixer taps allow this to be practised in safety in healthcare settings where water temperatures are high to combat *Legionella* spp.

4.80 Taps should be elbow-, knee- or sensor-operated (NHS Estates' HBN 4) for hand-wash sinks (see also "Hand-wash facilities" in "Isolation facilities" section, paragraphs 4.36–4.37).

4.81 Taps should be easy to turn on and off without contaminating the hands. Infrared taps are an alternative, but these are expensive (Bushell, 2000).

4.82 Taps discharging into a shallow sink or directly into a drain hole can cause splashing which disperses contaminated aerosols. Thus, the tap outlet flow should not point directly into the sink outlet (Ayliffe et al, 2000).

4.83 Avoid swan-neck tap outlets, as they do not empty after use. Strainers and anti-splash fittings at outlets should not be used as they easily become contaminated with bacteria.

Soap/disinfection dispensers

4.84 Skin antiseptics and soaps must be wall-mounted near the sink so that the user can operate the dispenser properly without risking contamination. Soap dispensers should not be refillable but be of a disposable, single cartridge design.

4.85 Alcohol-based hand cleaners have an important role, especially when access to hand-wash basins is difficult (Pittet, 2000). Unlike soap dispensers, these do not necessarily have to be placed by sinks.

Hand drying

4.86 Hand drying is of equal importance in maintaining hand hygiene as wet surfaces can transfer micro-organisms more effectively.

4.87 Paper hand-towels dry hands rapidly and dispensers can be used by several people at once. They are considered to be the lowest risk of cross-infection and are the preferred option in clinical practice areas (Bushell, 2000). The dispensers should be conveniently placed by hand-wash sinks.

4.88 The use of paper towels in rolls should be discouraged. They are difficult to tear off without contaminating the remaining roll (Gould, 1994; Hoffman and Wilson, 1994).

4.89 To discourage the use of reusable towels, towel rails should not be installed next to clinical hand-wash basins.

4.90 Fabric towels are recognised as a source of cross-contamination and are not recommended in clinical practice (Blackmore, 1987).

4.91 Hot-air dryers should not be used in clinical areas as warm air currents dry hands slowly and can be used by only one individual at a time. This results in queues and the temptation to dry hands on clothing (Bushell, 2000).

4.92 Foot-pedal-operated bins, with a waste bag, should be provided by each clinical wash basin (Gould, 1997).

Sinks and slop-hoppers

4.93 Using sinks for both hand-washing and the cleaning of equipment should be discouraged as this will significantly increase the risk of hand and environmental contamination (Finn and Crook, 1998); therefore, separate sinks should be installed for this purpose.

4.94 Separate sinks are required in sluice areas for the decontamination of bed-pan bases, wash bowls, etc. Where decontamination takes place, guidance provided by the Microbiology Advisory Committee (1999) must be adhered to.

4.95 Separate receivers such as slop-hoppers should be provided in areas where contaminated wastewater or blood and body fluids are disposed, i.e. dirty utility rooms and domestic store areas for cleaning equipment.

Recommendations

- A minimum of one hand-wash sink in each single room is required. En-suite single rooms should have a hand-wash basin in the en-suite facility in addition to a clinical hand-wash basin in the patient's room.

- Isolation rooms should have a hand-wash sink in the ante-room, isolation room and en-suite facilities.

- Ideally, in intensive care and high-dependency units (critical care areas), consideration should be given to providing one hand-wash basin at the front of each bed space (see NHS Estates' HBN 57: 'Critical care facilities'.

- In acute, elderly and long-term care settings, consideration should be given to providing one sink between four patients.

- In low-dependency settings, for example mental health units and learning disability units, consideration should be given to providing one sink between six patients

- In out-patient areas and primary care settings, a hand-wash basin must be close to where clinical procedures are carried out.

- Hand-wash sinks must be accessible and must not be situated behind curtain rails.

- All toilet facilities must have a hand-wash sink.

- The use of hand-wash sinks for purposes other than hand-washing must be discouraged.

- Wall-mounted cartridge soap/antibacterial agent dispensers and paper towels must be available at each hand-wash sink.

- Elbow-operated or non-touch mixer taps are required for all clinical hand-wash sinks.

- Hand-wash sinks must be designed for that purpose.

- Hand-wash sinks must not have a plug or overflow or be capable of taking a sink plug.

- The taps must not be aligned to run directly into the drain aperture.

- Waterproof splashbacks should be used for all sinks.

- Space must be allowed at the design stage for the placement of waste bins next to the hand-wash basin.

- Separate, appropriately sized sinks must be installed, where required, for decontamination. Two sinks will be needed: one for washing and one for rinsing, plus a hand-wash basin.

ANCILLARY AREAS

4.96 It is important that ancillary areas are of an acceptable standard and do not put the user at risk of cross-infection.

4.97 The evidence used is based on guidance from NHS Estates. Infection control issues will depend on:

- the use of the ancillary area;

- who will have access; and

- what type of activity will be carried out there.

4.98 Ancillary areas include:

- dirty utility/sluice;

- clean utility/SSD store;

- disposal room;

- day room/patient waiting areas;

- play areas;

- nappy-changing area;

- visitors' toilets;

- treatment room.

Dirty utility room

4.99 A dirty utility room should include facilities for:

- the cleaning of dressing trolleys and other items of equipment;

- testing urine;

- disposal of liquid waste; and

- temporarily holding items requiring reprocessing or disposal.

4.100 Space and facilities for holding and reprocessing of bed-pans, urinals and vomit bowls are required where in-patients are looked after (NHS Estates' HTM 2030). SSD returns can also be held here, along with storage of sani-chairs, commodes and linen bag carriers.

4.101 Hand-wash facilities are necessary plus the provision of a slop-hopper for disposal of body-fluid waste (NHS Estates' HBN 4 and HBN 36) and a separate deep sink for decontaminating nursing equipment.

Clean utility room

4.102 A clean utility room is required where drugs and lotions may be stored and prepared, a working supply of clean and sterile supplies may be held and dressing trolleys prepared. Clinical hand-wash facilities are required.

4.103 In primary care facilities, the room should be located adjacent to the treatment area. It is important that planners think about the type of storage facilities provided: there must be enough storage area for sterile supplies equipment and other clean supplies to keep supplies off the floor. They must be able to be cleaned easily and quickly while protecting clean stores and equipment from dust and contamination (NHS Estates' HBN 4 and HBN 36).

Treatment room

4.104 A treatment room may be required for in-patient examination or investigations on the ward. It will certainly be needed in primary care settings and will require different design features according to its planned use, for example immunisation, redressing or surgical intervention and investigations (NHS Estates' HBN 36).

- There should be enough hand-wash basins.

- Space should be available to allow for the storage of equipment and sterile supplies.

- Carpets should be avoided.

Disposal room

4.105 The disposal room is the temporary storage point for all items of supplies and equipment which have to be removed for cleaning, reprocessing or disposal for example linen, SSD items, waste disposal and sharps.

Day room/patient waiting areas

4.106 There is often conflict between the aesthetics of these areas and the prevention of contamination of the environment or furnishings. This is especially the case in waiting areas such as in accident and emergency departments, primary care and minor injury units (NHS Estates' HBN 4).

4.107 It is important that where blood and body-fluid spillages may occur, the environment should be able to be cleaned so that organisms do not survive.

4.108 Flooring should be cleanable and be able to withstand the use of detergents and disinfectants. Carpets are not recommended where spillage is anticipated.

Play area

4.109 There are infection control implications for toy cleaning (i.e. how they should be effectively cleaned) and storage (i.e. the provision of adequate toy storage facilities) plus issues for cleaning equipment and multiple use areas such as soft play areas and play mats (NHS Estates' HBN 36).

4.110 Porous or fabric toys should be avoided, as they cannot easily be decontaminated on site.

Nappy-changing area

4.111 Provision of a nappy-changing room is a necessary addition to any healthcare premises.

4.112 Facilities for disposal of soiled nappies and for hand-washing are required along with a regular cleaning programme of equipment used (NHS Estates' HBN 36).

4.113 The area for nappy-changing should have a surface that can be easily cleaned.

Visitors' toilets

4.114 These are heavily used and should provide enough space and have a high grade of finishes to maintain a good standard of hygiene.

4.115 There should be provision of disposal facilities for sanitary waste in both women's AND mixed-sex toilets.

4.116 The number of toilets and hand-wash basins provided must be sufficient for the anticipated population.

Recommendations

- Ancillary areas, provided as part of a ward, department, primary care facility or community home must be easily accessible, fit for the purpose and safe, both from a health and safety and from an infection control perspective.

- The infection control issues in an ancillary area must be included along with other design features and will depend on what the ancillary area is to be used for, who will have access and what type of activity will be carried out there.

- Ancillary areas must be easily cleaned, have facilities for hand-washing, disposal of fluid and clinical waste, if appropriate, and sufficient storage for supplies and equipment.

- Clean and dirty areas must be kept separate and the workflow pattern and management of each area must be clearly defined.

ENGINEERING SERVICES

4.117 Engineering services encompass areas where policy or procedural failure or emergencies could have wide-reaching and sometimes severe cross-infection implications for patients, staff or visitors.

4.118 This section discusses various aspects of engineering services and the infection control implications of each. Evidence is based on both guidance from NHS Estates and peer-reviewed papers. Areas discussed include:

- heating/temperature control;
- clean air and ventilation systems;
- hot and cold water systems;
- lighting;
- power and socket connections;
- patient power systems;
- wastewater and sanitation;
- medical gases.

Heating/temperature control

4.119 Special consideration should be given to the type of heating, cooling units and general ventilation systems provided in patient care and clinical areas.

Heat emitters (radiators)

4.120 NHS Estates' Health Guidance Note '"Safe" hot water and surface temperatures' provides guidance on how to prevent patients burning themselves on heat emitters.

4.121 The HGN recommends options to ensure safety as follows:

- guards/covers should be fitted;
- low surface temperature heat emitters should be used;
- flow temperature reduction (temperature controls fail to a safe position).

4.122 Of these options, covered heat emitters have raised the most infection control concern. Heat emitter covers allow dust to build up beneath and inside the heat emitter grille. This dust has been found to contain MRSA and other potentially pathogenic organisms, and when heat emitters are switched on during the winter months, dust and bacteria are dispersed by heat convection to the ward area.

4.123 Where heat emitter covers are used, regular planned maintenance and cleaning should be undertaken to prevent the problems described.

4.124 When installing heat emitters, it is recommended that there be adequate space underneath the heat emitter to allow cleaning machinery to be used. These areas may suffer from a lack of planned maintenance and cleaning and, as such, can become heavily contaminated with dust and potentially pathogenic organisms.

Pipework siting and access

4.125 "Hidden" heating may provide a solution to the problems of cleaning as long as access is possible for regular planned maintenance and cleaning. Pipework running externally along a wall can easily trap dust. External pipework to walls should be encased to facilitate easy cleaning.

Heating and general ventilation grilles

4.126 General heating/ventilation grilles need to be accessed easily for inclusion in cleaning programmes by domestic and estates staff. When infection outbreaks occur, it is essential that these fixtures and fittings are included in the cleaning process. Therefore, the ability for them to be easily removed and cleaned away from the patient area is essential in limiting cross-contamination. Cotterill et al (1996) and Kumari et al (1998) describe outbreaks associated with general ventilation grilles in an intensive care unit and an orthopaedic ward.

Heating and extraction ductwork

4.127 Heating and extraction ductwork should be installed in such a way that it can be accessed at fairly regular intervals and at frequent distances to limit cross-contamination.

Ceiling-mounted air-conditioning cassettes/units or air-conditioning wall-mounted units

4.128 These can be extremely difficult to clean, but because they can get very dusty, they should be installed with great caution and with the agreement for closure of the ward/department to enable satisfactory cleaning to be undertaken. Their use in high-risk areas can be problematic, as closure of these areas for cleaning is difficult.

Clean air and ventilation systems

4.129 Controlling airborne infection in relation to prevention of cross-infection in healthcare buildings remains a controversial subject. Hoffman et al (1999) divided the acute ward environment into:

- the "true environment", which comprises those organisms normally found in any non-hospital environment, for example fungal spores; and

- the "special hospital environment". This consists mainly of organisms arising from patients, staff and visitors, for example tuberculosis.

4.130 The relative incidence of airborne infection in hospitals has been estimated to be about 10% (Schaal, 1991); however, this does not take into account such factors as local respiratory pathogens, susceptibility of patients, climatic conditions, construction work, ventilation equipment and organisational policies in individual hospitals or wards.

4.131 The Control of Substances Hazardous to Health Regulations (COSHH) (1999) state that:

Exposure to a biological agent shall be adequately controlled by designing work processes and engineering control measures so as to prevent or minimise the release of biological agents into the workplace.

4.132 Thus, COSHH regulations require work processes to be safe by design; however, in some cases, such as multi-drug-resistant tuberculosis (MDRTB), both ventilation and personal protective equipment (PPE) will be required.

4.133 Shutters, access doors or air direction slats, if fitted, should be easily accessible for cleaning or removal.

Ventilation in the clinical setting

4.134 (For ventilation in isolation rooms, see "Isolation facilities" section, paragraphs 4.55–4.56.) Effective ventilation in healthcare premises involves the dilution of the airborne contamination by removing contaminated air from the room or immediate patient vicinity and replacing it with clean air from the outside or from low risk areas within the healthcare building. Engineering and planning of appropriate ventilation systems mainly relate to high risk units such as operating theatres, special care baby units, burns units, high dependency and intensive care units and areas such as isolation rooms (negative pressure ventilation for infectious patients and positive pressure ventilation for immunocompromised patients).

4.135 NHS Estates' HBNs and HTMs along with codes of practice for design of buildings give advice on natural ventilation, general extract ventilation and ventilation for specialist areas such as operating theatres, hydrotherapy suites, isolation rooms and are referenced under the respective specialist areas.

4.136 Research has suggested that in specialist areas, ventilation can reduce the incidence of healthcare-associated infection such as wound infections and communicable diseases (Ayliffe et al, 2000; Sanchez and Hernandez, 1999; Fox, 1997; O'Connell and Humphreys, 2000; Holton and Ridgway, 1993; Humphreys, 1993).

4.137 Wound infection has traditionally been a major cause of morbidity resulting from surgical procedures. Improvements such as ultra-clean theatre ventilation have contributed to reduced morbidity and mortality in specialist areas such as orthopaedics (Lidwell et al, 1982).

4.138 Airborne infections have been associated within treatment areas where patients are immuno-compromised, for example haematology wards, bone marrow transplant units (Alberti et al, 2001; Shererrtz et al, 1987).

Cost implications

4.139 In some clinical areas, the decision to install sophisticated ventilation systems which need routine or constant monitoring must be balanced against the risks and costs of such controls. The evidence on which to base the risk analysis is usually either absent or controversial. Where air movement is induced by mechanical ventilation, the flow of air must be from clean-to-dirty areas (where these can be defined). Hoffman et al (1999) state that "investment in mechanical air systems is large and as with many other areas of infection control, it is difficult to measure their true effectiveness when such a measure would be the absence of sporadic events implicating a failure of the system".

Control and containment of infection

4.140 Ventilation of healthcare premises is considered in NHS Estates' HTM 2025 and this includes discussion of airflow and filtration.

- Humphreys (1993) states that whenever airborne infection is possible in theatres, the airflow must go from clean to contaminated areas, and not the opposite way.

- Negative pressure facilities for airborne diseases are preferable.

- Isolation rooms can be equipped with appropriate ventilation, i.e. negative or positive airflow.

- Information on planned maintenance of ventilation systems should be available (see NHS Estates' HTM 2025: Vol. 4 – Operational management, pp 17–22).

- Ultra-clean ventilation systems in operating theatres can reduce airborne contamination and subsequent wound infections more effectively in specialist areas such as orthopaedics.

- Wagenvoort et al (1993) demonstrated the problems associated with intermittent interruption of electricity to ventilation systems which shuts the system down briefly.

Hot and cold water systems

4.141 Contamination of the water supply has been recorded as a cause of disease and death both in the public health arena and in the hospital setting. It is important, therefore, that drinking water in healthcare settings is safe, readily available to patients and is palatable to encourage drinking. The new EU Drinking Water Directive, which is transposed into UK law by the Water Supply (Water Quality) Regulations 2000, contains new provisions to ensure that the drinking water supply within buildings to which the public has access remains wholesome and is not adversely affected by the domestic plumbing system.

4.142 Access to chilled water may be important when patients are feeling unwell, pyrexial or the external temperature is rising. Patients who are ill become dehydrated and may need to increase their fluid intake.

4.143 A plentiful supply of water for other uses such as personal hygiene, hand hygiene and cleaning of the environment and equipment is also needed. Storage of this water requires careful consideration and can present problems if not dealt with appropriately.

4.144 Contamination of the water supply [for example *Legionella* spp. (Bartley, 2000)] can occur once it enters the building from the supply sources due to poor design of pipework, stagnation within pipes due to low usage, inappropriate storage or excessive cold water storage, or during renovation and refurbishment work.

Storage of water and policies for maintenance

4.145 Many organisms, such as species of non-tuberculous *Mycobacteria*, *Pseudomonas* and *Legionella*, have been isolated from hospital water systems. (For guidance on control of Legionella in water systems, see the Health & Safety Commission's (2001) guide: 'Legionnaire's disease: the control of Legionella bacteria in water systems'.) While some of these organisms are more likely to produce disease, many are potentially pathogenic. Problems have been documented in healthcare premises and are generally overcome by:

- cleaning water storage tanks;

- maintaining a consistently high temperature in hot water supplies or introducing a form of online disinfection (chlorine dioxide, ionisation) if lower temperature hot water is used to avoid thermostatic mixing valves and scalding (see Health & Safety Commission, 2001);

- regular maintenance of plant;

- removing dead-legs;

- keeping cold water systems cold; and

- minimising water storage.

4.146 In large hospitals, storage tanks are often necessary to ensure adequate supplies of water. Findings of *Aeromonas hydrophila* in seasonal trends by Picard and Goullet (1987) suggests that monitoring the water supply, especially during the summer months, is valuable. They also discuss the importance of keeping storage tanks clean and designing storage facilities to minimise excessive temperatures, which should then reduce the tendency for multiplication of not only *A. hydrophila* but also *Legionella* spp.

4.147 It is also good practice to ensure that hot and cold water pipework is separated (i.e. not in the same ducting) to avoid heat transfer to the cold water supply.

4.148 The need for testing is also raised following a survey of bacteriological quality of water from hospitals by Hunter and Burge (1988).

4.149 NHS Estates' HTM 2027 ('Operating policy') provides guidance on the monitoring and maintenance of water storage tanks.

Wash facilities

4.150 Showers are generally more acceptable to patients and the infection control team because of the difficulties of getting baths cleaned after each patient use, and there is potential cross-infection via this route. [Showers have been implicated in outbreaks of infection due to *Legionella* spp. (Tobin et al, 1980). Such problems, however, can be minimised by proper planned maintenance.]

4.151 WCs, bathrooms and showers should be designed and installed to aid cleanliness and prevent cross-contamination. Toilet facilities must have facilities for hand-washing and NHS Estates' HBN 4 recommends that they should be no more than 12 metres from the bed area or dayroom.

4.152 Claesson and Claesson (1995) documented an outbreak of endometritis in a maternity unit caused by spread of *S. pyogenes* (sometimes referred to as Group A streptococci) from a showerhead and their conclusion was that showers, when used to clean the perineum following childbirth, pose a definite risk for post-partum endometritis. Again, proper planned maintenance should minimise this risk.

Protection of patients with special needs

4.153 For areas with patients who have lowered immune responses, water fittings (washers, etc) should not support microbiological growth. Guidance can be sought from the Water Regulations Advisory Scheme (WRAS) (2001) 'Water Fittings and Materials Directory' and from BS 6920-1:2000 'Suitability of non-metallic products for use in contact with water intended for human consumption with regard to their effect on the quality of the water'.

4.154 Patients who have a lowered immune response are at risk from certain organisms found in water supplies in hospital and as such will need to be protected from this problem both in drinking water and washwater facilities. Steinert et al (1998) and Miyamoto et al (2000) discuss the effects of plumbing systems on *Legionella* spp. in hospital hot-water systems and methods of disinfecting.

4.155 Graman et al (1997) demonstrated how another outbreak of healthcare-associated legionellosis was traced to a contaminated ice machine. Wilson et al (1997) state that in the hospital environment, the greater proportion and range of susceptible individuals represent a high risk, borne out by the number of incidents of infection traced to hospital ice machines. Manangan et al (1998) produced guidance on the sanitary care and maintenance of ice-storage chests and ice-making machines in response to the problems and requests for guidance from infection control professionals. Guidelines where also produced by Burnett et al (1994).

4.156 In another incident with an ice-making machine, an MDA Hazard notice (Hazard (93) 42) was circulated following a report that leukaemia patients receiving chemotherapy treatment had developed septicaemia as a result of infection with *Stenotrophomonas maltophilia*. The source of this infection was traced to the storage cabinet of the ice-making machine in the ward. The notice gave guidance for immediate action to ensure that ice is made directly from water that is of drinking-quality.

4.157 Ice for the immunocompromised should be made by putting drinking water into single-use icemakers, then into a conventional freezer.

4.158 Bosshammer et al (1995) carried out comparative hygienic surveillance of contamination with *Pseudomonas* spp. in a cystic fibrosis ward over a four-year period and demonstrated how segregation of colonised and non-colonised patients was undermined through transfer of strains from a highly contaminated environment, that is, taps, sinks and wash basins.

4.159 Sniadack et al (1993) demonstrated how a pseudo-outbreak of *Mycobacterium xenopi* was attributable to exposure of clinical specimens to tap-water. This included rinsing of bronchoscopes with tap-water after disinfection; irrigation with tap-water during

colonoscopy; gargling with tap-water before sputum specimen collection and collecting urine in recently rinsed bed-pans.

4.160 Showers have been implicated in outbreaks of legionellosis in a transplant unit (Tobin et al, 1980) and on an alcoholism rehabilitation ward (Burns et al, 1991).

4.161 Water has been implicated in outbreaks not only from drinking water sources but also when it has been used for processing specimens, in equipment such as dialysis machines and as a contaminant in the environment and on hygiene facilities.

Lighting

4.162 Lighting levels should be maintained according to the recommendations for specific areas such as wards (day and night), theatres, corridors, examination rooms, ancillary or utility rooms and specific areas such as critical care units so that observation or patients is achieved without glare (HTM 2007). Additional task lighting needs to be provided in certain areas.

4.163 Location and design of luminaires should afford easy changing of lamps and frequent cleaning. They should be designed so that there are no ledges, ridges, etc., where dust can gather easily, build up and then be dispersed if the light is knocked or moved.

4.164 Light quality is as important as quantity and may help avoid mistakes such as invasive injuries during operative procedures or examinations.

4.165 Efficient lighting in all areas of wards or departments enables domestic staff to undertake cleaning more effectively.

Electrical power and socket services

4.166 Sufficient 13-amp switched and shuttered socket outlets should be provided in corridors and in individual rooms to enable domestic cleaning appliances with flexible leads (9 metres long) to operate over the whole department.

4.167 Where possible, socket outlets should be provided flush-mounted or in trunking systems to prevent the build up of dust.

Patient power system

4.168 The patient power (PP) system is a bedside entertainment and communication system that comprises a television and telephone. The patient uses a personal earpiece set for sound transmission. It is normally located on a flexible arm connection such that the patient can adjust it to achieve the best viewing position. An equipment box holding the electronics will, in most cases, be situated next to the bed.

4.169 System suppliers who have been approved by NHS Estates and are in possession of an NHS licence will have had the products evaluated and approved for use in the clinical environment and as such these products will **not** require special attention or cleaning.

4.170 The PP system should be cleaned on a regular basis as part of the normal bedside cleaning procedure. The specific manufacturer will advise on the precise nature.

4.171 The earpiece arrangement will have disposable foam pads, a supply of which should be readily available. Pads should be changed regularly, but always with a change of patient.

4.172 Decontamination, required after an incident, should be carried out in accordance with the manufacturer's instructions. These should be agreed by the Trust at the time the supplier is selected. Under no circumstances should liquid decontamination media be used without the manufacturer's instructions.

4.173 It remains the responsibility of the Trust to ensure that equipment is kept clean and compliant with infection control procedures.

Wastewater and sanitation

4.174 Domestic sewage contains a large number of intestinal organisms and is therefore hazardous. It must therefore be disposed of via a safe system internally to the external wastewater sewerage systems for treatment.

4.175 This waste will include water and body fluids from sanitaryware such as toilets and bidets plus drainage systems from mortuary tables and waste disposal systems and washer-disinfectors.

4.176 Wastewater is generated from a huge number of tasks carried out in healthcare buildings, which range from domestic cleaning, hand-washing, specialist laundries, surgical operations and areas such as renal dialysis units. Most of the wastewater contains micro-organisms from blood and body fluids and therefore has the potential for cross-infection if not disposed of safely.

Sanitary facilities

4.177 These not only include WCs and bidets but also equipment to assist patients who are unable to use a WC such as commodes and bed-pans, plus the equipment to disinfect this equipment such as bed-pan washer-disinfectors and macerators. The importance of cleaning in and around sanitary areas has also been shown in investigations of outbreaks caused by *Clostridium difficile* (Zafar et al, 1998; Cartmill et al, 1994. See also NHS Estates' 'National standards of cleanliness for the NHS').

4.178 Hospitals have recently seen increasing numbers of patients with *C. difficile*, vancomycin-resistant enterococcus (VRE) and diarrhoea and vomiting due to small round structured virus (SRSV). The degree of environmental contamination appears to be a determining factor in healthcare-associated infection, sanitary facilities acting as "hot spots" for transmission.

Internal drainage system

4.179 An internal drainage system must use the minimum amount of pipework, retain water and be air-tight at joints and connectors. It must be sufficiently ventilated to retain the integrity of water seals.

4.180 The design should comply with the relevant British Standards and Codes of Practice, including BS EN 12056 and the current building regulations. Recommendations for spatial and access requirements for public health engineering services are contained in CIBSE Guide G (Chartered Institution of Building Services Engineers, 1999).

4.181 Provision for inspection, rodding and maintenance should be located to minimise disruption or possible contamination and manholes should not be sited in clinical areas.

Waste disposal sinks

4.182 Sufficient and suitably located waste disposal sinks, for example sluice hoppers, should be provided to prevent contamination of hand-wash basins by disposal of wastewater.

Bed-pan washer-disinfectors/macerators

4.183 Where reusable bed-pans are used, ward areas require adequate and suitable bed-pan washer-disinfectors that comply with NHS Estates' HTM 2030 ('Washer-disinfectors'). Wards housing certain specialist areas, for example urology wards, will need more than one bed-pan washer-disinfector.

4.184 Individual assessment of need should be made; a uniform hospital policy will invariably mean some areas will be under-resourced. This also applies to the provision of macerators where disposable systems are used. Where macerators are used, there should be facilities to wash-disinfect bed-pan holders.

4.185 Rutala and Weber (1999) detail the role of disinfection and sterilization and discuss sanitary equipment in what they term "non-critical item decontamination". With the emergence of VRE as a healthcare-associated pathogen during the past five years, urine containers and bed-pans have been implicated in outbreaks (Bonten et al, 1996).

4.186 Control or containment of these outbreaks depends on many factors, but not least the safe disposal of wastewater and sanitation and cleanliness of the equipment/environment.

4.187 Where fitted, bed-pan washer-disinfectors should be installed according to the Water Supply (Water Fittings) Regulations 1999 to prevent backflow and contamination.

Medical gas vacuum systems

4.188 Vacuum and suction equipment is a potential cross-infection risk. The delivery system is similar to that of gases, i.e. piped or via mobile equipment. The vacuum pipe system must be able to be isolated in case of incidents where pipework becomes contaminated with blood/body fluid. Contamination of piped vacuum delivery systems can cause problems for estates personnel. Access to the pipework may involve removal of the wall fabric and ceiling. The use of vacuum-controlled units with overflow protection devices is essential to avoid contaminating the system with aspirated body fluid. Instructions for cleaning are given in NHS Estates' HTM 2022 'Operational management'. Instructions for bacterial filter change are also contained in this document.

4.189 HTM 2022 gives guidance regarding piped medical gases and vacuum systems and includes recommendations on:

- emergency procedures;

- power failure;

- access for cleaning contaminated vacuum systems;

- training and communication;

- maintenance and infection risk.

4.190 Before carrying out any maintenance work on vacuum systems and/or changing bacterial filters, the infection control team should be informed so that advice can be given on any appropriate precautions to be observed.

Recommendations

- Heat emitters should be designed and installed in a manner that prevents build-up of dust and contaminants.

- Heat emitters, heating and general ventilation grilles should be easily accessible for cleaning.

- Ventilation should dilute airborne contamination by removing contaminated air from the room or immediate patient vicinity and replacing it with clean air from the outside or from low-risk areas within the healthcare building.

- Lighting should be planned so that lamps can be easily cleaned, with no ledges or ridges where dust can gather.

- The use of vacuum-controlled units with overflow protection devices for mechanical suction is essential to avoid contaminating the system with aspirated body fluid.

- Contamination of the water supply can occur due to poor design of pipework, inappropriate storage or during renovation and refurbishment work. Such problems can be overcome by:

  - cleaning water-storage tanks;

  - maintaining a consistently high temperature in hot-water supplies or introducing a form of on-line disinfection (chlorine dioxide, ionisation) if lower temperature hot water is used to avoid thermostatic mixing valves and scalding (see Health & Safety Commission, 2001);

  - maintaining plant regularly, minimising dead-legs;

  - keeping cold water systems cold; and

  - minimising water storage (NHS Estates' HTM 2027 and HTM 2040).

- Protection of patients with special needs: patients who have a lowered immune response are also at risk from certain organisms found in water supplies in hospital and will need to be protected from this problem with particular attention to drinking water and washwater facilities.

- Ice for the immunocompromised should be made by putting drinking water into single-use icemakers, then into a conventional freezer.

STORAGE

4.191 (For the storage of **clinical waste**, see the "Waste – segregation, storage and disposal" section, paragraphs 4.276–4.304.)

4.192 Storage is required for bulky items of equipment, as well as smaller items used in the clinical setting, to protect them from dust or contamination. The need for sufficient storage should not be underestimated.

4.193 This section discusses the need for storage areas in healthcare settings and the rationale for appropriate provision for equipment, patient personal possessions and waste/linen.

4.194 Areas discussed include:

- the importance of access for cleaning;

- patient-centred storage;

- design;

- storage during construction;

- quantity;

- large equipment.

The importance of access for cleaning

4.195 The role of the environment and environmental decontamination in preventing cross-infection has been discussed by several authors (Talon, 1999; Cartmill et al, 1994). It has been difficult to prove cause and effect due to the multitude of factors involved, but recent studies have increasingly implicated the environment in the spread of healthcare-associated infection. Disposable items delivered in bulk restrict cleaning access if not appropriately stored.

4.196 Bacteria such as *Staphylococcus aureus* have been shown to survive in dust on equipment for long periods (Duckworth and Jordens, 1990; Hirai, 1991). Equipment, therefore, should be stored in appropriate storage areas to reduce contamination.

Patient-centred storage

4.197 Patients need lockers or wardrobes for storage of their personal possessions and clothing. These pieces of furniture are frequently missed in the cleaning process following discharge of patients. Louvre doors should not be fitted as they are difficult to keep clean and they have been shown to harbour dust containing pathogenic organisms.

Design

4.198 The type of storage facility needs consideration. In practice, storage racks, boxes and shelves need to be accessible and cleaned quickly and easily. Thought given to the type of racking or storage system purchased will reduce cleaning input in the long term. Lack of cleaning due to time constraints leads to potential reservoirs of cross-infection in storage areas. This is particularly hazardous where clean equipment or sterile supplies are being stored.

4.199 There must be enough storage space to keep equipment and supplies off the floor. Shelving should be low enough to discourage this; yet, it should also be high enough to enable cleaning underneath the bottom shelf.

Storage during construction

4.200 Clinical areas must maintain appropriate storage areas during construction, which may be difficult because of lack of space. Temporary storage must be clean, maintain appropriate temperature and humidity control and should be free of pests (Carter and Barr, 1997).

Quantity

4.201 Many plans start with storage areas built in to the design, but often clinical staff and designers do not appreciate the importance of these areas and if extra space is required take these designated areas for other purposes. This then leads to problems when clinical activities begin and can have implications for both clinical practice and health and safety.

Large equipment

4.202 There is a need for the provision of a large storage area within all healthcare premises to enable the storage of large pieces of equipment such as beds, mattresses, hoists, wheelchairs and trolleys that are required but not currently in use. The use of equipment libraries has become a more cost-effective way of not only storing large or electrical equipment, but also maintaining and cleaning this equipment in a more controlled way.

4.203 Many trusts struggle to store such equipment following new builds, because the issue has been ignored during the design and planning stage of development. This then causes problems due to lack of dedicated space. The associated infection control risk is that equipment stored in corridors and around bed spaces prevents adequate cleaning.

Recommendations

- Patients need lockers or wardrobes for their personal possessions and clothing.

- Domestic cleaning equipment, laundry and clinical waste need to be stored in separate purpose-built areas to prevent cross-contamination (see also "Laundry and linen services" and "Waste – segregation, storage and disposal" sections).

- All healthcare premises need a storage area for large pieces of equipment such as beds, mattresses, hoists, wheelchairs and trolleys which are not currently in use.

- Sufficient and appropriate storage will not only protect equipment from contamination and dust which may potentially carry micro-organisms but also allow free access to floors and shelves for domestic cleaning.

FINISHES AND FLOORS, WALLS, CEILINGS, DOORS, WINDOWS, INTERIOR DESIGN, FIXTURES AND FITTINGS

4.204 Guidance on the selection of finishes is provided in NHS Estates' HBNs and HTMs pertinent to the area that is being planned, that is, catering department, operating theatre, etc. The quality of finishes in all areas should be of a high standard so that there is ease of cleaning and the fabric of the building stays intact. Cost allowances in HBNs make due recognition of this need. It is important that the healthcare environment is aesthetically pleasing but takes into account the nature of the intended purpose.

4.205 This section discusses:

- hard flooring in clinical areas;

- carpets;

- finishes;

- fixtures and fittings;

- walls;

- ceilings;

- doors;

- windows;

- soft furnishings;

- curtains and blinds (window and bed);

- radiators;

- work surfaces.

Hard flooring in clinical areas

4.206 Flooring should be smooth, easily cleaned and appropriately wear-resistant.

4.207 There should be coving between the floor and the wall to prevent accumulation of dust and dirt in corners and crevices.

4.208 Any joints should be welded or sealed where they are unavoidable. Sealing prevents damage due to water ingress under the flooring.

4.209 Attractive impervious flooring materials (such as vinyls) are readily available. This provides a surface that can be easily maintained and cleaned.

4.210 Flooring must be properly anchored, as lifting of the flooring material can create a reservoir for infectious agents.

4.211 Wood and unsealed joints and tiles must be avoided as they may produce reservoirs for infectious agents (Bartley, 2000).

4.212 In areas where frequent wet cleaning methods are employed (for example clinical areas and theatres), floors should be of a material which is unaffected by detergents and disinfectants.

4.213 Floors subject to traffic when wet (bathrooms, kitchens) should have a non-slip surface.

Carpets

4.214 Carpets should be avoided in ALL clinical areas. This includes all areas where frequent spillage is anticipated (Bushell, 2000; Ayliffe et al, 1999). Spillage can occur in all clinical areas, for example, ward areas, clinics, single rooms, corridors and entrances. Aesthetic considerations are most often cited as the reason for using carpets; yet, in areas of frequent spillage or heavy traffic, they can quickly become unsightly. Problems of smell and staining have been responsible for the removal of carpets in many clinical areas. It would seem preferable to avoid carpets in these areas as attractive alternatives are available (Ayliffe et al, 1999).

4.215 Carpets are associated with retention of odour, particularly in facilities where there is body-fluid spillage. They may also be damaged by chlorine-releasing agents used for decontamination of blood and body fluid spillages and during outbreaks of infection. Carpets are therefore considered unsuitable for areas where body-fluid spillage frequently occurs and also where food and drink frequently cause soiling, ultimately resulting in odour problems (Bushell, 2000).

4.216 Washable floors rather than carpets are also advisable in isolation/single rooms as carpets may prolong the survival of certain organisms [for example, MRSA (Ayliffe et al, 1999)].

4.217 There is a growing body of evidence suggesting that carpets do become contaminated and can be associated with outbreaks of infection:

- a study of bacterial contamination of floors and other surfaces in operating rooms identified the highest colony counts in dressing rooms, the floors of which were covered with carpets and cleaned with a vacuum cleaner (Suzuki et al, 1984);

- Cheesbrough et al (1997) reported an outbreak of illness in two male carpet-fitters due to small round structured virus (SRSV), which was not related to contaminated food. The most likely source of infection was the carpet;

- Sarangi and Roswell (1995) identified that high numbers of *Streptococcus pyogenes* (sometimes referred to as Group A streptococci) were present in carpets and soft furnishings during an outbreak. Steam-cleaning was required to significantly reduce the numbers of these micro-organisms;

• carpets have been shown to be heavily contaminated by *Clostridium difficile* (Skoutelis et al, 1994).

4.218 If carpets are purchased, it is essential that in addition to buying suitable carpets (carpets with impervious backing are available) and cleaning equipment, the cleaning schedules are agreed upon before the carpet is bought and that they are achievable. The cleaning guidelines provided by manufacturers are often impractical because they may require evacuation for the procedure.

4.219 Facilities should also be available for the prompt removal of spillage over a 24-hour period (Ayliffe et al, 1999).

Finishes

4.220 Materials and finishes should be selected to minimise maintenance and be compatible with their intended function. All finishes in clinical areas should be chosen with cleaning in mind, especially where contamination with blood or body fluid is a possibility (i.e. smooth, non-porous and water-resistant).

4.221 Design should ensure that surfaces are easily accessed, will not be physically affected by detergents and disinfectants and will dry quickly. Building elements that require frequent redecoration or which are difficult to clean or service should be avoided (NHS Estates' HBN 4).

4.222 Wall surfaces should also be free from fissures, open joints or crevices that may permit retention of dirt/dust and insects. Floors or walls penetrated by pipes, ducts and conduits should be sealed tightly to stop entry of rodents and insects.

Fixtures and fittings

4.223 Fixtures and fittings should be accessible for cleaning. If they are not cleaned on a regular basis, they may be potential reservoirs of infection. The environment has been implicated in cross-infection and organisms such as MRSA, *Clostridium difficile* and *Acinetobacter* spp. are of increasing importance.

4.224 Equipment that is in direct contact with patients has been implicated in infection outbreaks (Irwin et al, 1980). Equipment that is within the immediate patient environment has been shown to be a potential source of cross-infection. Fixtures and fittings, if difficult to access or clean on a regular basis, fall into this category and must be included as a potential reservoir of infection when risk assessment is undertaken. Design should

ensure that surfaces are easily accessed, will not be physically affected by detergents and disinfectants and will dry quickly.

4.225 Modular furniture (self-assembly) that is not easily moved should be installed on raised platforms, or suspended in some manner to achieve a minimum 6–12 inches clearance from the floor so that they can be pulled out for cleaning, or so that they can be cleaned underneath (Bartley, 2000).

Walls

4.226 Smooth, hard, impervious surfaces are recommended in clinical areas as they are easier to clean and bacteria cannot readily adhere to them (Bartley, 2000; Ayliffe et al, 1999). Design should ensure that surfaces are easily accessed, will not be physically affected by detergents and disinfectants and will dry quickly.

Ceilings

4.227 Smooth, hard, impervious surfaces are recommended in theatres and isolation rooms. Caution should be used when considering the use of ceilings to produce visually appealing areas, as they can be difficult or time-consuming to access for cleaning, for example hidden lighting or box-work.

4.228 False ceilings may be associated with accumulation of dust or fungi and can harbour pests. It is therefore essential that buildings are checked on completion to ensure that no unwanted materials from the building works remain and that there is no access for pests (Ayliffe et al, 1999). Ceilings with removable tiles or perforated ceilings can allow dust to fall onto the area below during maintenance work. This type of ceiling should therefore be avoided in isolation rooms, operating theatres and treatment rooms (Ayliffe et al, 1999). See also NHS Estates' HTM 60.

4.229 Pipes and cables running through walls above false ceilings should be sealed so far as is reasonable.

Doors

4.230 All bays and single rooms require doors if they are to be used for cohort barrier nursing or isolation nursing. They should have smooth handles which can be easily cleaned, will not be physically affected by detergents and disinfectants and will dry quickly (see NHS Estates' HTM 58).

Windows

4.231 Windows, although not directly an infection control issue, allow patients in isolation to feel less shut off from the world and have been shown to add to the therapeutic process when a pleasant view can be seen.

4.232 Glass partitions, instead of solid walls, enable patients to see what is happening in the ward but there will also be a need to allow for patient privacy at times. Double-glazed windows with integral blinds are practical and solve all cleaning problems.

4.233 Windows should be fixed and sealed in operating theatres, treatment rooms and isolation rooms.

4.234 Avoid ledges as in cottage-style windows because this will allow for the accumulation of dust; ledges also require a significant cleaning commitment. (See NHS Estates' HTM 55 and HTM 56.)

Soft furnishings

4.235 Soft furnishings (for example, seating) used within all clinical and associated areas should be covered in a material that is impermeable. Fabric that becomes soiled and stained cannot be adequately cleaned and so may require replacement (Noskin et al, 2000). Again, design should ensure that surfaces:

- are seam-free where possible;

- can be accessed easily for cleaning;

- will not be physically affected by detergents and disinfectants; and

- will dry quickly.

Curtains and blinds (windows and bed)

4.236 Curtains have been shown to become easily contaminated with staphylococci and streptococci and remain contaminated for months (Palmer, 1999). These micro-organisms can be transmitted by hand to patient by touching the curtain.

4.237 Curtains can be laundered and this must be carried out **at frequent intervals** to reduce contamination by micro-organisms. A policy needs to be developed locally for the regular laundering of curtains and for changing curtains that become contaminated or used near patients with communicable infections. All curtains purchased must be able to withstand washing processes at disinfection temperatures (71°C for three minutes or 65°C for ten minutes).

4.238 Venetian blinds are not recommended, because they become dusty and are extremely difficult to clean. If used in specialist areas, such as theatres or ophthalmic departments, they should be enclosed between glass. Washable and detachable blinds can be used, but it is difficult to clean them as frequently as curtains and, thus, usually need specialist cleaning contracts. Roller-blinds, if used, should also be enclosed between glass.

4.239 The use of dividers or screens that can be manoeuvred on wheels can be of benefit in ITU areas.

The use of these dividers requires consideration at the planning stages as extra space is required both for their use between beds and for storage. It is important that they are easily cleanable.

Radiators

4.240 Radiators have also been implicated in outbreaks of infection with MRSA and are often difficult to clean because they are enclosed in bay windows or in protective covers to prevent burns. They should be smooth, accessible and cleanable.

4.241 Pipework should be contained in a smooth-surfaced box that is easy to clean; pipework sited along a wall can become a dust trap and can be impossible to clean.

4.242 Pipes and cables running through walls above false ceilings should be sealed so far as is reasonable.

Work surfaces

4.243 Surfaces should be designed for easy cleaning.

4.244 Surfaces near plumbing fixtures should be smooth, non-porous and water-resistant.

4.245 They should be free of fissures, open joints and crevices that will retain or permit the passage of dirt particles.

4.246 All joints must be sealed (Bartley, 2000).

4.247 Horizontal surfaces can become contaminated. Therefore regular cleaning is required.

4.248 All surfaces must be able to withstand regular cleaning with both detergent and disinfectant products.

Recommendations

- The quality of finishes in all areas should be of a high standard and cost allowance in HBNs makes due recognition of this need. Guidance on the selection of finishes is provided in several HTMs.

- Soft furnishings must be covered in an impervious material within all clinical and associated areas.

- Flooring should be smooth, easily cleaned and appropriately wear-resistant.

- The use of carpets is NOT advised within any clinical or associated area. Attractive vinyl flooring materials are available which can provide aesthetic appeal.

- All joints and crevices should be sealed.

- Curtains must be able to withstand washing processes at disinfection temperatures.

- Window blinds should be used with caution; the need for regular cleaning in clinical areas must be considered.

- All surfaces should be designed for easy cleaning.

- Smooth, hard, impervious surfaces should be used for walls.

- All surfaces, fittings, fixtures and furnishings should be designed for easy cleaning and durability.

DECONTAMINATION

4.249 The effective decontamination of medical devices is essential in reducing the risks to patients from healthcare-associated infection and minimising the potential iatrogenic transmission of TSEs, that is, Creutzfeldt–Jakob Disease (CJD), variant Creutzfeldt–Jakob Disease (vCJD), Gerstmann–Sträussler–Scheinker Disease (GSS) etc.

4.250 Decontamination is the combination of processes which include cleaning, disinfection and sterilization used to render a reusable medical device safe for re-use on patients and for handling by staff. This section discusses the importance of decontamination of medical devices and the evidence which can be used as a useful checklist for planning areas in the built environment that are included in the decontamination "life-cycle" shown in Figure 2.

4.251 Each of the segments represents a stage in the decontamination process. At all stages, consideration should be given to location, facilities, equipment, management and policies/procedures.

4.252 Areas discussed in this section include:

- decontamination and healthcare-associated infection;

- transmission of vCJD;

- decontamination assessment tools;

- decontamination facilities and accommodation.

Healthcare-associated infection

4.253 It has been demonstrated that 10% of in-patients have a hospital-acquired infection (now referred to as healthcare-associated infection) at any one time, the most common being urinary tract infection, surgical wound and lower respiratory tract infection.

4.254 There are common risk factors which cause infection, but it is not known how many infections could be prevented by improving decontamination procedures; however, it is known that failure in decontamination processes can result in a range of infections. Saksena et al (1999) reported that transfer of infectious material had been demonstrated in inadequately decontaminated instruments. Medical Devices Agency, Hazard Notice HN 9503, May 1995, referred to water contaminated with *Pseudomonas aeruginosa* being used to flush the lumens of a microsurgical hand-piece, which

Figure 2 Decontamination life-cycle of reusable surgical instruments

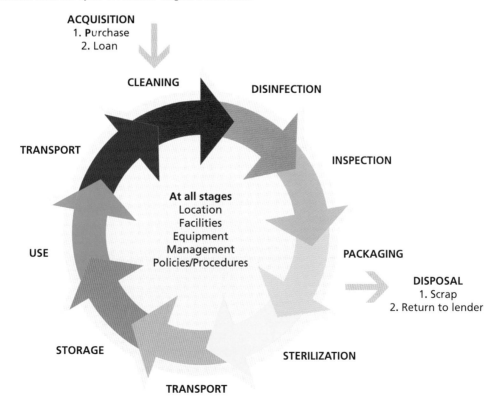

subsequently suffered ineffective sterilization before use. Three patients who had undergone surgery at the same time were found to be infected.

4.255 Therefore, effective decontamination can make a contribution to preventing healthcare-associated infection, and this is best achieved if facilities are "planned in" for the process to be achieved during the full "life-cycle" of decontamination of medical devices.

Transmission of vCJD

4.256 The possibility that vCJD might be spread from person to person in healthcare situations may arise for a number of reasons:

- classical CJD has been transmitted from person to person by medical procedures;

- abnormal prion protein has been demonstrated in the lymphatic tissue (including tonsils) of patients with established vCJD;

- abnormal prion protein has been demonstrated in the appendix of a patient who subsequently developed vCJD;

- abnormal prion protein may not be inactivated by normal sterilization procedures.

4.257 Research which gave rise to these concerns includes the identification of the abnormal form of prion protein reported in the appendix removed from a patient some months before he went on to develop clinical signs of vCJD (Hilton et al, 1998). This was the first time that the presence of abnormal prion protein had been detected in peripheral tissues before the onset of clinical disease. Furthermore, in another study (Hill et al, 1999), lymphoreticular tissues (tonsils, spleen and lymph nodes) from patients with neuropathologically confirmed vCJD were found to be positive for the abnormal protein associated with prion diseases.

4.258 The Spongiform Encephalopathy Advisory Committee (SEAC), which advises the Government on BSE/CJD issues, has advised that rigorous implementation of washing, decontamination and general hygiene procedures are key measures in reducing the risk of vCJD transmission via surgery. A risk assessment model, developed by the Department of Health at SEAC's request and published in March 2001, confirms this ('Risk assessment for transmission of vCJD via surgical instruments', available on the DH website at http://www.doh.gov.uk/cjd/riskassessmentsi.htm).

Decontamination assessment tools

4.259 Following a snapshot survey of decontamination methods and facilities in healthcare premises in England (1999/2000), immediate and medium-term actions where set out in Health Service Circular 2000/032: 'Decontamination of Medical Devices'. This was to allow a more comprehensive survey of decontamination provision across the NHS to take place. Organisations were provided with the 'Decontamination Programme Technical Manual – Part 1: Process Assessment Tool and Decontamination Guidance' (Department of Health, 2001).

4.260 This tool provides the mechanism for an organisation-wide review of decontamination facilities and services. It assesses compliance against relevant Department of Health guidance, including provision of sterile supply service accommodation. There are elements within the process assessment tool that can be used to assess the provision of existing local reprocessing areas including suitability of storage arrangements, transport cleanliness and staff training.

4.261 The 'Decontamination Programme Technical Manual – Part 2: Decontamination Organisational Review Information System (DORIS)' (Department of Health, 2001) allows organisations who have used the process assessment tool to evaluate the information collected and to model their service delivery profiles.

Decontamination facilities and accommodation

4.262 If decontamination is to be undertaken in a safe and effective manner that reduces risk and contributes to a reduction in healthcare-associated infection, then it must be carried out in a suitable environment, with validated automated processes, managed and operated by trained staff.

4.263 Centralised reprocessing of surgical instruments is the preferred option and local reprocessing should be the exception rather than the norm. Accommodation provided for decontamination should be designed and operated in a manner that does not contribute to the overall bio-burden of the instruments being processed. NHS Estates' HBN 13 provides advice and guidance on provision of central sterile supply accommodation. Where local provision is required then it must be carried out to the same standard as central reprocessing.

4.264 The Microbiology Advisory Committee (1999) manual 'Guidance on Decontamination' gives advice on implementing reprocessing procedures. There is a local decontamination protocol (Department of Health 2001, http://www.doh.gov.uk/decontaminationguidance/decon.pdf) for use where centralisation is not a viable alternative in the short term. Of particular note to infection control staff is the provision of separate sinks for washing and rinsing of instruments in addition to designated sinks for washing of hands. Segregation of clean and dirty decontamination processes also has implications for preventing spread of infection.

4.265 When designing clinical accommodation, consideration should be given to providing adequate and appropriate storage for centrally provided sterile supplies. If sterile supplies are stored inappropriately, then sterility can be compromised and contamination can occur.

Recommendations

- In order to review elements in the built environment which impact on decontamination of surgical instruments and other reusable medical devices which are invasive by intent, it is necessary to look at the whole life-cycle of surgical instruments.

- The process assessment tools in the 'Decontamination Programme – Technical Manual' act as a useful checklist for planning areas in the built environment which are involved in purchasing, processing, maintaining, storing and using medical devices.

- Local reprocessing should be the exception rather than the norm and, therefore, facilities should be designed with adequate and appropriate storage for centrally provided sterile supplies.

LAUNDRY AND LINEN SERVICES

4.266 Laundry from hospitals and healthcare establishments may be contaminated with blood or body fluids and may have been used on infected patients. It must be disinfected during the washing process to prevent the risk of infection to both patients and staff. Standards lower than those which can be obtained in a commercial machine should not be accepted without full consideration of the risks (Ayliffe et al, 1993). Large quantities of laundry can only be dealt with effectively in large industrial washers and tumble dryers [Barrie, 1998; Department of Health, HSG 95(18)].

4.267 Used linen should be segregated at source into three categories and bagged appropriately before sending to the laundry:

1. used linen

2. heat labile linen

3. infected linen (which should be placed onto either a water soluble liner or a bag with a water-soluble membrane before placing it into the laundry bag).

4.268 Policies must be in place to inform staff of the segregation procedure for the three types of linen to ensure that there is safe practice for all those involved in the handling and decontamination "chain" [Department of Health, HSG 95(18)].

4.269 There should be separate storage areas for both clean linen and the storage of linen awaiting collection or laundering (NHS Estates' HBN 4).

4.270 Processing of heat labile garments may be required and the use of a low temperature wash and hypochlorite will be required for this purpose [Department of Health, HSG 95(18)].

4.271 There is a need to separate used, heat labile and infected linen from clean linen (NHS Estates' HBN 25). Staff working in a large laundry may be provided with different coloured uniforms to discourage them from moving from one area to another.

4.272 Thermal disinfection is required and is achieved by holding the wash temperature for three minutes at 71°C or ten minutes at 65°C. Appropriate machines are therefore important and the equipment must be monitored and calibrated regularly.

4.273 Staff must have easy access to a hand-wash basin and possibly a shower in the event of a spillage, accident or contamination. Staff must be alerted to the possible risk of mishap from extraneous items that are accidentally included with the soiled linen. Infection of laundry staff has rarely been reported (Standaert et al, 1994), but suitable protective clothing, correct procedures and provision of an occupational health service will be necessary.

Recommendations

- Linen has to be disinfected during laundering and rendered free of vegetative pathogens. In this way, prevention of infection to both patients and staff is achieved.

- Large quantities of linen produced in healthcare establishments can only be dealt with effectively in large industrial washers and tumble dryers.

- In both hospitals and the laundry, there should be separate storage areas for clean laundry and used laundry which is awaiting collection or decontamination.

- Used linen should be divided at source into three categories (used linen, heat labile linen and infectious linen) and bagged in appropriately colour-coded bags before sending to the laundry.

- There is a need to carefully segregate used linen from clean linen in commercial laundries or launderettes. The work should flow from dirty to clean areas. Consideration should be given as to whether different coloured uniforms should be supplied to discourage staff from moving from one area to another.

- Where launderettes are provided in hospitals for long-stay patients, the following areas should be considered:

    1. The infection control department must be involved in the planning and design of any new launderettes.

    2. The area to be used must be specifically designated as a launderette and no other activities must be carried out there, for example eating or smoking.

    3. The walls and floor must be washable and internal decoration must be to an acceptable standard.

    4. Washers and dryers of an industrial standard must be purchased (domestic washing machines have a very small rinse cycle). Washers must have a sluice and disinfection cycle and dryers must be vented to outside.

    5. The machines should be sited on a plinth so that pumps can be omitted. (These are a potential cross-infection risk.)

    6. There must be segregation of clean and dirty linen and sufficient storage facilities for both.

    7. There must be provision of a separate hand-wash basin and all necessary protective clothing such as gloves, aprons etc.

- Washing machines must incorporate temperature-recording equipment which is regularly monitored and calibrated.

- There must be appropriately sited hand-wash basins in sufficient quantity and with easy access for staff.

- Staff changing rooms and sanitary facilities should be provided for male and female staff. There must be access to a shower room.

- Infection control teams should be included in the review and auditing of healthcare contracts.

CATERING/FOOD HYGIENE

4.274 Ill patients can be particularly vulnerable to the effects of food-borne infection. This is usually traced to a bacterial source and problems can arise from food handlers, utensils and work surfaces as well as incorrect or inadequate food hygiene precautions. It is important that management control systems [for example HACCP (Hazard Analysis and Critical Control Points): see the Department of Health's (1993) 'Assured safe catering – a management system for hazard analysis'], good

practices and the conditions in which the food is stored, prepared, processed, distributed and served all enable high standards of hygiene to be achieved and readily maintained.

4.275 To facilitate appropriate standards of personal hygiene for staff, there should be hand-wash basins in each preparation area and in the cooking and serving areas. Non-touch taps should be specified, and liquid soap and paper towels should be provided. Basins should be sited where they cannot splash onto food preparation equipment.

Recommendations

- All healthcare establishments must comply with the food safety requirements in the Food Safety Act 1990 and food hygiene regulations made under this Act.

- There are many requirements when planning or upgrading a new catering facility. The Department of Health's 'Health Service Guidelines: management of food hygiene and food services in the NHS' and 'Hospital catering: delivering a quality service' both give useful guidance. Initial planning and design meetings should include the local authority environmental health inspector, key managers and the infection control team.

- When deciding on the location of the building, it is important to remember that there will be regular deliveries to the kitchen from outside suppliers. It is essential that delivery vehicles can gain easy access and catering staff are able to monitor the delivery temperature and unpack and store the food quickly. Similarly, there must be prompt distribution of food trolleys from the kitchen to the serving areas.

- A first consideration should be to establish the type of catering that will be provided, for example the regeneration of frozen food will require different facilities from those needed for the preparation of fresh food.

- The facility must be large enough to cater for the number of meals and the type of food production.

- The layout, design and construction must be designed to ensure that high standards of cleaning and disinfection can be maintained. The finishes to walls, floors, work surfaces and equipment must be capable of withstanding regular cleaning and the impact of mechanical cleaning equipment.

- There must be separation of the processes for handling raw and cooked food and separation of "clean" and "dirty" activities (food preparation and dishwashing).

- Food preparation areas must be physically separated from the store for the cleaning equipment and from sanitary facilities.

- There should be adequate facilities for the safe storage, at correct temperature, of raw, fresh and cooked frozen foods. It may be necessary to include cooling rooms/larders for controlled cooling before refrigeration, blast chillers for rapid cooling, thawing cabinets for controlled thawing, chilled vegetable stores, chilled service units, ice-making equipment and heat lamps over bains-marie.

- It must be possible to be able to monitor the correct temperature of a process from equipment used (for example that dishwashers achieve thermo-disinfection).

- An adequate number of suitably located hand-wash basins must be provided.

- Each hand-wash basin and every sink provided must have an adequate supply of hot and cold water.

- Drains must be adequate for the purpose.

- The ventilation must be sufficient to maintain a comfortable environment for the staff and prevent the premises and equipment from overheating. Artificial ventilation systems must be constructed to permit access for cleaning and maintenance. Condensation will encourage the growth of mould.

- Precautions should be taken to prevent the entry of insects, rodents and other pests into any area of food storage or preparation.

- The disposal of food waste must be separated from the food preparation area and be pest and rodent proof. A water supply and floor-level drainage is required to deal with spillages and for cleaning.

- Staff toilets and changing rooms with showering facilities should be provided (HBN 10).

- Ward kitchens, pantries and therapeutic kitchens: equipment purchased must conform to the standards in the Food Safety Act and regulations under the Act. This includes the need for a separate hand-wash basin and finishes used for the floors, walls, etc. The size and design will vary according to the overall decision for food preparation in the premises. If a cook-chill system or regeneration of frozen food is to take place, the kitchen will need to be larger to house the regeneration oven and will need additional ventilation.

- The reprocessing of crockery and cutlery is achieved more effectively with a central dishwashing facility in the hospital setting.

WASTE – SEGREGATION, STORAGE AND DISPOSAL

4.276 There are stringent legislative controls and clear working guidelines for the management of healthcare waste and good design can minimise problems with waste segregation, storage and disposal.

4.277 This section discusses the problems of waste management and the guidance that must be adhered to if patients, staff and contractors are to be protected. The reality is that the disposal of waste is often poorly managed and inadequately catered for in wards, departments and community healthcare establishments and this can lead to escalating costs and heightened risks to healthcare staff.

4.278 Following a study of hospital waste management on 13 hospital sites, the Audit Commission (1997) stated that on average an acute hospital of 500 beds produces over 10 tonnes of waste a week. Some of the waste such as paper, food scraps, flowers and bottles is disposed of into the household waste stream and costs between £20 and £70 per tonne. The rest consists of clinical waste and special waste and costs considerably more to dispose of – between £180 and £320 per tonne.

4.279 Areas discussed include:

- identification/segregation;

- disposal/clinical bins;

- hospital waste;

- community waste;

- construction waste;

- final disposal;

- clinical implications.

Identification/segregation

4.280 Identification of categories and the means of segregation of clinical and special waste form the key elements of a waste disposal strategy. Waste is a risk not only to healthcare staff but also to their colleagues, patients, visitors and contractors. Increasing costs, litigation and damage to the environment are also areas for concern.

4.281 The means of segregation will depend on the ratio of clinical waste to non-clinical waste. Space at the ward/unit level is needed for suitable waste containers, whether the area served produces large or small amounts of clinical waste and household waste. Bins must be supplied in the appropriate areas according to amounts produced.

4.282 Current strategies and future strategies for clinical waste management are outlined in NHS Estates' HTM 2065 along with the present legislative and regulatory framework and guidance.

4.283 The Audit Commission (1997) report also contains an overview of waste management strategies.

4.284 Blenkharn (1995) discusses the disposal of clinical waste and the development of more recent waste treatments.

4.285 Hooper (1994) outlines one hospital's method of waste minimisation and discusses the possible environmental impact.

Disposal/clinical bins

4.286 Clinical bin lids sustain the heaviest bacterial contamination and need to be capable of being suitably cleaned and disinfected (Ayliffe et al, 1993). Therefore, the use of bins with a removable body to allow for adequate cleaning is recommended.

4.287 Bins should be foot-operated only, and the foot pedal should be sturdy and durable. A bin mechanism that cannot be opened by hand – but only by a foot pedal – is the ideal.

Hospital waste

4.288 Storage trucks in hospital streets (corridors) have been used for clinical waste. However, as a result of the NHS Plan (http://www.nhs.uk/nationalplan/) and PEAT (patient environment action teams – http://www.nhsestates.gov.uk/property/peat_content.html) work, it has been suggested that these trucks are unsightly and should be removed. Therefore, any new developments must allow for disposal storage cupboards sited at the entrance to the ward or department, preferably with access from both ward and hospital street. Waste can then be stored in this area – instead of cluttering up dirty utility rooms, which are often inadequate – while awaiting collection by the portering staff.

4.289 These can be combined with soiled linen and household waste, but must be clearly subdivided so that the three types of waste are separated from each other. This will assist rapid collection and should minimise the risks of items for reprocessing being accidentally taken for disposal by incineration.

4.290 The subdivided areas must be able to be cleaned in the event of spillage and must be able to contain any

spillage that does occur. The hold area should be large enough to hold a wheelie-bin, which in turn would reduce handling and the subsequent risks to the porters. A designated, secure collection bay is also necessary to hold bins until waste is either incinerated/compacted/treated on-site or transported off-site for incineration (Audit Commission, 1997; Health Services Advisory Committee and the Environment Agency, 1999; NHS Estates' Health Guidance Note, 1995; Spencer, 1997).

Community waste

4.291 In healthcare facilities such as nursing/residential homes and primary care settings, all waste must be contained in bags inside a lockable container to comply with appropriate guidance (Health Services Advisory Committee and the Environment Agency, 1999).

4.292 The system and frequency of collection of waste service for the particular area needs to be taken into account when planning facilities needed for temporary holding bays, etc. If located externally, the holding bay or bin must be washable, secure and rodent-proof.

4.293 There must be a strict routine for removing waste to ensure it does not remain uncollected for extended periods.

Construction waste

4.294 Each year, 70 million tonnes of waste are produced by the construction industry and for projects attached to existing healthcare facilities this can cause considerable risk to highly susceptible patients. It is important that this dust and debris is controlled and disposed of safely.

4.295 Barrier systems must be erected and closed waste containers supplied.

4.296 Traffic control through designated entry and exit areas and dedicated lifts should be identified, if possible.

4.297 Keys et al (2000) outline the problems arising from waste produced by the construction industry and suggest that to remove waste you have to design it out.

Final disposal

4.298 Space at the ward/unit level is needed for provision of suitable waste containers, whether the area served produces large or small amounts of clinical waste. The storage facilities provided will vary with type of healthcare facility and method of final disposal.

4.299 This is mainly achieved by the use of commercial, high temperature incinerators capable of meeting the increasingly tight emission limits set out by UK regulations.

4.300 Under the Environmental Protection Act 1990, certain types of clinical waste such as body parts and chemicals must be incinerated at high temperature. However, much of what is usually designated as "clinical waste" does not necessarily have to be burned, but must be rendered safe.

4.301 Current strategies and future strategies for clinical waste management are outlined in NHS Estates' HTM 2065 along with the present legislative and regulatory framework and guidance. The Audit Commission report (1997) also contains an overview of waste management strategies.

4.302 Introduction of large-scale alternatives have so far been limited, but given the pace of new technological change and changing regulations it is important at the design and planning stage of any new build that consideration is given to new methods that may emerge. These methods of disposal of clinical waste may provide a more cost-effective or greener option for the future.

Clinical implications

4.303 The clinical implications that arise when the system for managing waste in healthcare goes wrong or is simply not in place are:

- risks to staff/patients from contamination and cross-infection from blood and body fluid;

- invasive injury and subsequent risk of acquiring blood-borne viruses for patients, staff and the general public;

- risk from incorrectly segregated pharmaceutical waste and cytotoxic waste;

- risk from incorrectly bagged radioactive and laboratory waste;

- risk to immunocompromised patients from incorrect transporting and disposal of construction waste.

4.304 The current legislation governing clinical waste disposal and what happens when the regulatory guidelines are breached is outlined by Moritz (1995). Evidence is lacking that most clinical waste, other than perhaps sharps or waste from patients with certain infectious diseases, is a significant hazard to the public. Phillips (1999) states that more still needs to be done in this area of risk management and also in proving the efficacy of alternative processes for its management.

Recommendations

- Systems in place must be capable of protecting patients, staff, contractors and the environment from harm.

- The risk of invasive injury and contamination by blood and body fluids increases if waste is not segregated/stored and disposed of correctly. Cost and risk are therefore the prime motivation for improvements in primary waste disposal practice and for the provision of facilities in the built environment to accomplish it.

- Storage/disposal hold: the storage facilities provided will vary with type of healthcare facility and method of final disposal.

- Future strategies will need to include green issues in disposal of clinical waste.

CHANGING FACILITIES

4.305 Facilities should be provided for staff not only to encourage them to change out of their uniform in the workplace but also to be able to store their personal effects safely. Patients also need changing/storage facilities. Hand-wash basins and shower facilities for staff should be provided in the event of blood or body fluid splashes.

4.306 This section discusses the need for changing facilities for staff and patients and the key elements to consider:

- design and quantity;

- out-patient changing areas;

- staff changing areas;

- sanitary facilities;

- type of uniform provided;

- distance from clinical areas.

Design and quantity

Out-patient changing areas

4.307 In areas such as out-patients, imaging and minor injuries units, it will be necessary to provide changing/storage facilities if clothing has to be removed and kept safe. These should be included at the planning stage and must be able to be cleaned easily.

Staff changing

4.308 By providing staff changing facilities, staff will be able to change from hospital or unit uniform into outdoor clothes on-site. In practice, this will deter staff from travelling home in their uniform.

4.309 Showers should be provided in case of splashes, spillage with blood or body fluid. Hand-wash basins should also be provided to encourage hand-washing after changing. The distance from the working area may dictate how frequently staff use the facilities.

Maintenance staff

4.310 Consideration should also be given to providing changing facilities for maintenance staff, service engineers, etc., who may have to change into theatre gowns and overshoes for work carried out, for example, in clean utility rooms.

Sanitary facilities

4.311 Separate staff changing rooms, sanitary facilities and showers should be provided for male and female staff with sufficient locker space for outdoor clothing and personal effects.

Type of uniform

4.312 The type of uniform and laundry facilities may dictate the type of facilities needed.

Recommendations

- Changing facilities should be provided for staff to encourage them to change out of their uniform in the workplace. They will also need to be able to store their personal belongings safely while on duty.

- Hand-wash basins and sanitary facilities should be included, and showers should be provided in the event of contamination by blood or body fluid.

SERVICE LIFTS/PNEUMATIC DELIVERY SYSTEMS

Service lifts

4.313 Healthcare premises depend on lifts to provide an efficient, fast and segregated vertical transport system for the movement of patients, staff, visitors, medical equipment and ancillary services.

4.314 Lifts are categorised according to their use. In healthcare premises, they fall into one of the following categories:

- passenger lift;

- bed lift;

- goods lift.

Passenger lift

4.315 Pedestrian traffic is defined as all ambulant people who require transportation between floor levels (staff, patients and visitors). The location of out-patient departments, day surgery and similar departments

generating large numbers of ambulant people should therefore be identified.

Beds lift

4.316 The need to move high dependency patients in beds with equipment may arise if hospital design includes wards such as critical care units which are not on the same level as theatres.

Goods lift

4.317 There is a constant flow of food, clean/soiled linen, drugs, sterile supplies etc, which is essential to the smooth operation of a hospital.

Recommendations

- It is important during a planning stage and when refurbishment work is to be undertaken to remember that hospitals have their own unique traffic patterns. These will vary according to the nature of the departments being served, relative locations of lift entrances, links to other buildings and the type of patients/staff/visitors using the areas.

- In some locations, traffic groups can be segregated to optimise on efficiency, degree of urgency and to provide some degree of privacy for patients, that is, theatre traffic, accident and emergency traffic or high-dependency patients.

Pneumatic-air tube transport systems

4.318 Pneumatic-air tube transport systems provide an effective, rapid and secure means of transporting various items such as blood and tissue samples, drugs, imaging films and documentation from one department to another.

4.319 The advantages of this system of transport for the laboratory are:

- faster turn-around time for specimens;

- automated computer-assisted forms;

- service available 24 hours a day.

4.320 The disadvantages are:

- may have limited capacity – large specimens may still need to be delivered in other ways;

- risk of infection/cross-infection;

- reduced security/error in labelling.

4.321 The safe use of pneumatic-air tube transport systems is fundamentally reliant on:

- types of specimen suitable for dispatch;

- the design, notably of the specimen carrier and network of tubing;

- giving staff the right information and training so that proper operating and control procedures are always followed;

- the tubes themselves being segregated for pathology, pharmacy and imaging.

4.322 The use of pneumatic-air tube transport systems for the delivery of microbiology samples including blood culture bottles presents no problems in sample quality and improves the timeliness of specimen arrival (NHS Estates' HTM 2009).

4.323 The number of lost or mislaid specimens has been shown to be reduced under this system.

Breakage or spillage of samples

4.324 Spillage within the tube should be a rare occurrence if the system is being used in a safe manner and staff have received the appropriate training. Any high risk samples should be placed in a leak-proof container which in turn is placed in a sealed plastic bag incorporating a request form.

Recommendations

- The carrier for specimens should be transparent, able to be autoclaved and incorporate a leak-proof seal.

- If leaking samples are allowed to enter the tube system or station, the station should be isolated and dealt with following advice from the infection control team. The disinfection procedure or cleaning will depend on the nature and level of risk imposed by the contaminant. Each incident will need to be assessed separately.

- Major policy decisions with reference to the system should be made through the infection control committee.

DESIGN FOR A CLEAN, SAFE ENVIRONMENT

4.325 The importance of a clean, safe environment should not be underestimated. It is important that healthcare buildings are designed with appropriate finishes and fittings that enable thorough access, cleaning and maintenance to take place. Good standards of basic hygiene, cleaning and regular planned maintenance will assist in preventing healthcare-associated infection. If the built environment reflects these needs, schedules are more likely to be successfully undertaken on a proactive and reactive basis.

4.326 This section discusses evidence and rationale for best practice relating to a clean, safe environment from which recommendations are made.

4.327 Areas discussed include:

- ward housekeepers;

- hotel services and estates departments;

- patient perspective;

- the role of the environment in cross-infection;

- design for cleaning and maintenance;

- finishes, fittings and furniture;

- radiators and ventilation systems;

- storage;

- prompt removal of obsolete equipment;

- adequate lighting and provision of power sockets for cleaning;

- provision of suitable cleaning equipment;

- planned preventative maintenance/refurbishment;

- IT equipment.

Ward housekeepers

4.328 The introduction of a new post – that of ward housekeeper [NHS Plan, 2000 http://www.nhs.uk/nationalplan/; see also 'Housekeeping' by NHS Estates (2001)] – will assist the ward manager in making sure that the ward and medical equipment is kept clean and that the environment is properly maintained. This should have positive effects on the prevention of cross-infection.

Hotel services and estates departments

4.329 Cleaning in high-risk areas where organisms can accumulate on high-tech equipment or in areas that are difficult to access due to design, such as behind pipework, is equally important in preventing the spread of infection.

Patient perspective

4.330 It is difficult to evaluate a healthcare building from a patient perspective. It is considered that the institutional feel of some facilities do little to reduce patient anxiety. Poor lighting and poor colour schemes can exacerbate patient unease (Miller and Swensson, 1995).

4.331 There is sufficient evidence to implicate the patient environment as a potential reservoir of infection and, therefore, measures to minimise and control this contamination should be inclusive in the planning and design stages of healthcare buildings. It is important to note that the aesthetic appeal of the environment and the psychological needs of the patient are important areas to consider in the planning process.

The role of the environment in cross-infection

4.332 Recent studies have suggested that bacteria can exist and survive for long periods in the hospital environment (Duckworth and Jordens, 1990; Musa et al, 1990; Hirai, 1991; Smith et al, 1998; Talon, 1999) with furniture, fixtures and fittings acting as reservoirs of infection. This may increase the risk of cross-infection.

4.333 In studies carried out by Boyce et al (1997) and Talon (1999), evidence showed that a contaminated environment was implicated in the spread of healthcare-associated infection with multi-resistant bacteria.

4.334 Rampling et al (2001) demonstrated how extra attention to the environment and cleaning schedules resulted in the reduction of infections in a surgical environment; however, audit of cleaning by visual inspection is also failing to highlight problem areas (Griffith et al, 2000).

4.335 It has been suggested that the level of domestic and general cleaning has decreased in recent years (ICNA/ADM, 1999). While equipment has become more complex and difficult to clean, healthcare facilities have not always been designed with infection control in mind.

Design for cleaning and maintenance

4.336 If healthcare buildings are designed in such a way as to facilitate easier access for cleaning and maintenance, it is more probable that these processes will be carried out effectively within the limited time available.

4.337 Infection control teams agree that maintaining good standards of hospital hygiene is a cost-effective method of controlling healthcare-associated infections and that improved cleaning standards are achievable (Dancer, 1999). Cleaning schedules must be robust.

4.338 During prolonged outbreaks, it may be advisable that the environment be microbiologically, as well as visually, monitored.

Finishes, fittings and furniture

4.339 These should be easily cleaned and sufficiently robust to withstand the prolonged use of disinfectants such as chlorine-releasing agents or alcohol-impregnated wipes.

Radiators and ventilation systems

4.340 The lack of planned cleaning programmes for these areas results in layers of dust and bacteria accumulating with the potential for spread of infection.

4.341 These areas are often difficult to access and estates departments have had to prioritise their resources in line with decreasing budgets. Hospital directorates or the internal market system need to be aware that they need to request and pay for this service or they will not be carried out.

Storage

4.342 Lack of adequately sized storage facilities for large pieces of equipment and the consequent inappropriate siting of such equipment and other general items make it difficult to gain access for cleaning.

Prompt removal of waste and obsolete equipment

4.343 Appropriately designed disposal areas and agreed systems for the disposal of this type of equipment allows for prompt removal, which in turn enhances cleaning programmes.

Adequate lighting and provision of power sockets for cleaning

4.344 Both of these items are essential if cleaning is to be undertaken to a high standard.

Provision of suitable cleaning equipment for clean finishes

4.345 Suitable equipment must be provided for the type of finishes and furniture provided. Areas such as theatres and critical care will need specialist cleaning expertise.

4.346 Accommodation must also be provided where cleaning equipment can be cleaned and stored. This facility should include a slop-hopper sink for disposal of potentially contaminated cleaning water.

4.347 Hand-washing facilities are also required.

Planned preventative maintenance/refurbishment

4.348 There are many areas that are not accessible for routine, daily cleaning and which will need specialist knowledge or equipment to access. In such circumstances, the estates department has an important role to play in the cleaning of equipment/facilities, such as vents, grilles, catering equipment, hydrotherapy pools and high-level cleaning in theatres.

4.349 Planned cleaning programmes need to be discussed and agreed so that they are instigated on a regular basis. For critical care areas, theatre suites, sterile services departments, catering and laundry, planned preventative maintenance is crucial for the smooth operation of these services. Any untoward event in any of these areas can have severe and disastrous infection control implications.

4.350 Before maintenance or refurbishment of clinical areas begins, managers, ward staff, the estates department, hotel services and members of the infection control team need to collaborate to minimise risk and disruption.

IT equipment

4.351 IT equipment collects dirt and dust – which contain micro-organisms with the potential for cross-infection – if not cleaned regularly and properly. In clinical areas, alcohol wipes can be used to remove dust.

Recommendations

- Areas to consider are:

  - surfaces that facilitate easy cleaning (smooth, hard, impervious floor finishes, benches, walls and ceilings);

  - welded/sealed joints to prevent water egress;

  - sealed skirting boards;

  - low dust retention fixtures/fittings;

  - splash-backs to sinks and in-tact seals around sinks;

  - adequate storage facilities for equipment not in use;

  - bed storage/cleaning facilities;

  - storage for cleaning equipment;

  - adequate supplies of equipment and PPE;

  - colour-coded segregation of cleaning equipment;

  - communication and time to clean additional areas such as isolation rooms/bays involved in outbreaks;

  - induction and regular in-service training.

- Accommodation must be provided where cleaning equipment can be cleaned and stored. This facility should include a slop-hopper sink for disposal of potentially contaminated cleaning water. Hand-washing facilities are also required.

CONSTRUCTION AND THE ROLE OF CLEANING

4.352 Construction inevitably generates dirt and, with it, certain micro-organisms that potentially may harm immunocompromised patients [especially *Aspergillus fumigatus* (see Appendix 1)]. Dust and debris control is crucial in tandem with the need for increased and regular cleaning during and after completion of the building project. Bartley (2000) discusses the role of infection control and reviews the environmental dispersal of micro-organisms during construction. Infection control teams should be involved in discussions before external cleaning contracts are awarded (see Appendix 6).

4.353 This section discusses evidence and rationale for best practice relating to the control of dust and debris from construction work from which recommendations are made.

4.354 Areas considered include:

- refurbishment/new build;

- workflow;

- infection risk/patient movement;

- specialist areas – theatres, critical care, laundry, treatment areas.

Refurbishment/new build

4.355 Standards set out in NHS Estates guidance documents essentially apply to new buildings. However, the principles therein should be applied as far as possible where existing accommodation is being upgraded (summary of principles – see Appendix 6).

Workflow

4.356 Correct workflow systems must be maintained throughout the building project. Infection control teams need to be guided by the design team and collaboration between the two teams and appropriate advice must be sought during the planning of specialist units such as theatres and critical care so that these principles are not compromised.

4.357 Most departments have clean-to-dirty-area flow systems so that staff can practice safely. Workflow is at the heart of basic infection control practice when the built environment is being considered. There is often an issue of space "being at a premium" and often the temptation is to fit everything in somehow.

Recommendations

- A planned cleaning programme is essential when building work of any nature is planned.

- Workflow and agreed time-scales are important to prevent incidents that potentially put patients/ clients at risk.

- Frequent auditing (visual and microbiological) of the area involved will highlight any problems.

- Early involvement of the infection control team in the planning process will alleviate potential infection control risks.

Appendix 1 Description of some infectious agents linked with healthcare-associated infections

Name of organism/ genus	Type of organism/ transmission	Further information	Population affected	Epidemiological factors
Aspergillus fumigatus	A ubiquitous fungus, spore-forming. Airborne (inhalation); also contact transmission reported.	Bartley (2000); Cornet et al (1999); Manuel and Kibbler, (1998); Mahieu et al (2000); Richardson et al (2000); Thio et al (2000)	Bone marrow transplant, haematological malignancies with prolonged neutropenia for example acute leukaemia	Increased risk during construction and renovation. Reservoirs of *Aspergillus fumigatus* include soil, dust, bird droppings, building materials, window air-conditioners/filters, false ceilings, tiles, humidified cell incubators, lifts, carpeting, air filter replacements
Bacillus cereus	A Gram-positive, spore-forming bacillus	Dancer (1999)	At-risk patients. Associated with food poisoning, but also non-gastrointestinal cases recorded in maternity, surgical and ICUs	Association with building work
Clostridium difficile	Anaerobic, Gram-positive bacillus	McCulloch (2000); Dancer (1999)	Older adults, children	Spores may survive for months on furniture, toilets etc, contaminated hands, equipment or in the environment
Klebsiella spp.	Gram-negative bacillus	Dancer (1999)	At-risk patients	Known to survive well on surfaces. Once a reservoir is established, the organisms may be transferred to patients directly or indirectly, generally by hands
Legionella spp.	Gram-negative bacteria. Waterborne, spread by inhalation of aerosol. May cause Pontiac fever and legionnaires' disease	Brundrett (1992); Bartley (2000); NHS Estates' HTM 2040; Dobson et al (1997) all discuss engineering design; McCulloch (2000)	All age groups may become infected, most susceptible are patients with serious underlying diseases. Men typically affected more than women (2:1), and higher between 40 and 70 years of age. (Brundrett, 1992). May progress to pneumonia	Soil, water, cooling towers; water storage tanks, infrequently used showers. Optimum growth for *Legionella* spp. at 35–37°C although environmental isolates grow best around 30°C.
Mycobacterium xenopi	Waterborne	Bartley (2000)	Endoscopy	Water, scopes
Penicillium spp.	Airborne	Bartley (2000)	Bone marrow transplant	Rotted wood cabinet, ventilation ducts, fibreglass insulation
Pseudomonas paucimobilis	Waterborne	Bartley (2000)	ICU	Water used to fill flush water bottles
Methicillin-resistant *Staphylococcus aureus* (MRSA)	Gram-positive bacterium. Environmental contamination contact. Can withstand desiccation and is thus a frequent component of hospital dust	McCulloch (2000); Dancer (1999); Report of a combined working party on the control of MRSA (1998); Wagenvoort et al (2000)	Endemic in hospitals and the wider community. At-risk patients	Methicillin-resistant *Staphylococcus aureus* (MRSA) has penetrated virtually every hospital and a chronic endemic state remains in most, with episodes of cross-infection and outbreaks. *S. aureus* has been isolated from the knobs of TVs, cushions, computer keyboards, pens, curtains, bedding, nurses' uniforms

Name of organism/ genus	Type of organism/ transmission	Further information	Population affected	Epidemiological factors
Small round structured virus (SRSV), for example Norwalk virus	Faecal–oral and airborne as evidenced by explosive nature of outbreaks	Kaplan et al (1982)	High attack rates >50% in outbreaks among children	Faecal shedding 0 to 72 hrs and infectivity at +2 and +3 days
Vancomycin-resistant enterococcus (VRE)	Human and animal gastrointestinal tract, persists in its host long-term	Dancer (1999)	In at-risk patients, vancomycin-resistant enterococci (VRE) sepsis is extremely difficult to treat	More resistant to disinfectants, survives well in hospital environment; no effective regimens to clear human carriage
Verocytotoxin-producing *Escherichia coli* (VTEC)	Gram-negative bacillus	McCulloch (2000)	Children, older adults – may lead to renal failure	Environmental sources are many and varied. Good food hygiene, hand and environmental hygiene. Exclude from work affected food handlers.

Appendix 2 Infection control risk assessment during construction/refurbishment of a healthcare facility

1. First, identify **construction activity type** from the table below.

Type A	Inspection and non-invasive activities, includes, but not limited to: • removal of ceiling tiles for visual inspection on corridors and non-clinical areas; • painting and minimum preparation in corridors and non-clinical areas; • electrical trim work (all plugs, switches, light fixtures, smoke detectors, ventilation fans); • minor plumbing and activities that do not generate dust or require cutting of walls or access to ceilings other than for visual inspection.
Type B	Small scale, short duration activities that create minimal dust. Includes: • removal of a limited number of ceiling tiles in low risk clinical areas for inspection only; • installation of telephone and computer cabling; • access to chase spaces; • cutting of walls or ceiling where dust migration can be controlled in non-clinical areas.
Type C	Any work of long/short duration which generates a moderate-to-high level of dust or requires minor building works, demolition or removal of any fixed building components or assemblies. Includes, but is not limited to: • sanding of walls for painting or wall covering; • removal of floor coverings, ceiling tiles, panelling, and wall-mounted shelving and cabinets; • new wall construction; • minor duct work or electrical work above ceilings; • major cabling activities.
Type D	Major demolition and construction projects. Includes, but is not limited to new construction/machinery and equipment installations, rectifications and modifications

2. Then identify the **infection control risk group** by area.

Group 1 (low risk)	Group 2 (medium risk)	Group 3 (high risk)
Office areas/corridors plant rooms/ service ducts	A&E clinical rooms Radiology/magnetic resonance imaging General surgery recovery units Wards Nuclear medicine Admissions/discharge units Echocardiography Other departmental clinical areas Out-patient department Pharmacy (general) Laboratories Hydrotherapy pools Endoscopy clinics Examination rooms	Day surgery rooms All intensive care units All operating suites All high dependency units Dialysis & transplant units Oncology Cardiology Cardiac catheterisation suite Pharmacy clean rooms Sterile Services Departments

3. Now identify the "risk class" by correlating "construction type" with "risk group" (from 1 and 2 above) in the matrix below.

	Construction activity type			
Risk group	**Type A**	**Type B**	**Type C**	**Type D**
Group 1	Class 1	Class 2	Class 2	Class 3
Group 2	Class 1	Class 2	Class 3	Class 3
Group 3	Class 2	Class 3	Class 3	Class 4

4. After identifying the risk class from 3 above, follow the risk measures advised for each class.

Class 1	• Execute work by methods to minimise dust from construction • Immediately replace any ceiling tile displaced for visual inspection
Class 2	• Where appropriate, isolate HVAC (heating, ventilating, and air conditioning) system in areas where work is being performed • Provide active means to prevent airborne dust from dispersing into atmosphere if practicable, i.e. dust bag to machine • Water-mist work surfaces to control dust while cutting • Avoid pooling of water which may be prolonged • Seal unused doors with duct-tape • Block off and seal air-vents • Wipe work surfaces with detergent • Contain construction waste before transport in tightly covered containers • Wet-mop and vacuum with filtered vacuum cleaner before leaving work area • Place dust-attracting mat at entrance and exit of work area (tacky mat) • Remove isolation of HVAC system
Class 3	• Where appropriate, isolate HVAC system in area where work is being done to prevent contamination of duct system • Complete all critical barriers and implement dust control methods before construction begins • Maintain negative air pressure within work site. Use HEPA (high efficiency particulate air)-equipped air filtration unit if there be a risk that air will enter building • Do not remove barriers from work area until complete project is clinically clean • Vacuum with filtered vacuum cleaner during works • Wet-mop area during works • Remove barrier materials carefully to minimise spreading of dust and debris associated with construction • Contain construction waste before transport in tightly covered containers • Remove isolation of HVAC system in areas where work has been done and appropriate checks performed
Class 4	• Isolate HVAC system in area where work is being done to prevent contamination of duct system • Complete all critical barriers and implement dust control methods before construction begins • Maintain negative air pressure within work site using HEPA-equipped air filtration unit • Seal holes, pipes, conduits and punctures appropriately • Construct airlock and require all personnel to remove dirty apparel and clean down before leaving the work site. The use of cloth/paper disposable overalls/shoes, etc., may be required • Do not remove barriers from work area until completed project is thoroughly cleaned (as before) and repeat clinical clean after barrier removed • Vacuum work area with filtered vacuum cleaner • Wet-mop area with detergent during works • Remove barrier materials carefully to minimise spreading of dust and debris associated with construction • Contain construction waste before transport in tightly covered and sealed containers • Remove isolation of HVAC system in areas where work has been done and appropriate checks performed

Appendix 3 The capital investment process

Figures 1–3 are from Appendix 2 ("The capital investment process") of the "Overview" booklet of the 'Capital Investment Manual'. (Note: the 'Capital Investment Manual' is currently being rewritten.)

Figure 1 Components of the 'Capital Investment Manual'

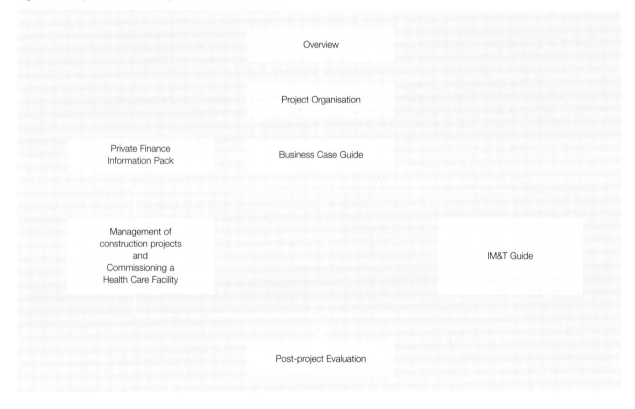

Overview

Project Organisation

Private Finance
Information Pack

Business Case Guide

Management of
construction projects
and
Commissioning a
Health Care Facility

IM&T Guide

Post-project Evaluation

Figure 2 The capital process for health buildings and equipment

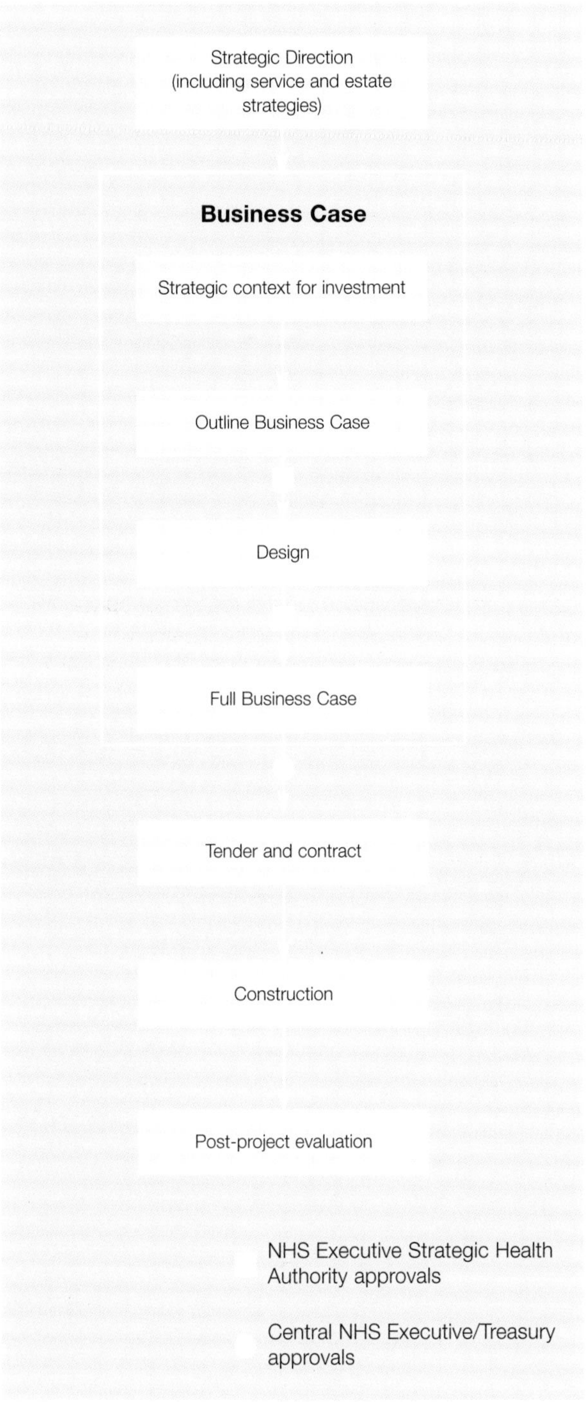

Strategic Direction
(including service and estate strategies)

Business Case

Strategic context for investment

Outline Business Case

Design

Full Business Case

Tender and contract

Construction

Post-project evaluation

NHS Executive Strategic Health Authority approvals

Central NHS Executive/Treasury approvals

Figure 3 Capital investment process for private finance

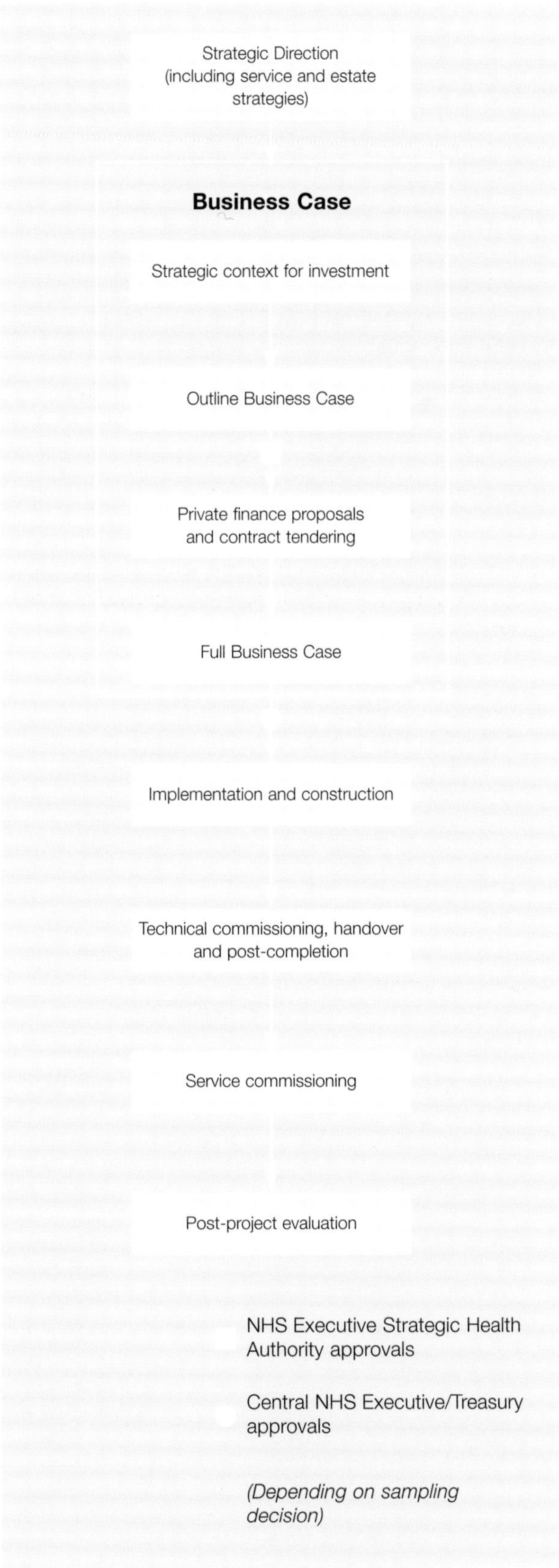

Strategic Direction
(including service and estate strategies)

Business Case

Strategic context for investment

Outline Business Case

Private finance proposals and contract tendering

Full Business Case

Implementation and construction

Technical commissioning, handover and post-completion

Service commissioning

Post-project evaluation

NHS Executive Strategic Health Authority approvals

Central NHS Executive/Treasury approvals

(Depending on sampling decision)

Appendix 4 Equipment groups

Equipment supplied for new building schemes can be in one of four categories.

Items which are supplied and fixed under the terms of a building/engineering contract and funded within the works cost. These are generally large items of plant/equipment which are permanently wired/installed, that is:

1. excluded from this group will be items subject to late selection due to considerations of technical change, for example radiodiagnostic equipment

2. specialised equipment items best suited to central purchasing arrangements

Taps and basins also fall into group 1 equipment.

Group 1 items are specified at the design stage.

Items which have implications in respect of space/construction/engineering services and are installed under the terms of building engineering contracts, but are purchased by the Trust under a separate equipment budget, for example:

- paper towel dispensers;
- soap/scrub dispensers;
- cupboards;
- shelving;
- washer-disinfectors;
- washing machines;
- worktops.

Items which have implications in respect of space and/or construction/engineering services and are purchased and delivered/installed directly by the trust, for example:

- small refrigerators;
- furniture;
- ventilators;
- monitors;
- trolleys.

Items which may have storage implications but otherwise have no impact on space or engineering services, for example surgical instruments.

Appendix 5 Notification of capital project

NOTIFICATION OF CAPITAL PROJECT

**to Fire Advisor/Security Advisor/H&S Advisor/Infection Control Team/Microbiologist/
Risk Management/Estates/Hotel Services/IT/Telecomms/RRPPS**

Scheme title

Location

Job no.

Project Manager

Date

Current stage ☐ concept ☐ brief ☐ design ☐ tender ☐ on site

Approx. start

Approx. value

Brief description of works

The work involves:	limited amount	extensive
Work in or near a clinical area	☐	☐
Noisy work adjacent to patient areas	☐	☐
Dusty work adjacent to patient areas	☐	☐
Work to H&C water services	☐	☐
Air-conditioning/ventilation	☐	☐
Asbestos removal	☐	☐
Imaging/lasers	☐	☐
New data and telephone outlets	☐	☐
(Other)	☐	☐

Architect

M&E designer

Planning Supervisor

User Representative

Appendix 6 Summary of principles and approach to infection control in capital planning projects

1. Draw up and agree Policy prior to commencement of work to include:

- Gantt chart to outline expected timescale for:

    - patient area closure as appropriate (who is responsible?);

    - isolating air handling units (plumbing) (who is responsible?) services;

    - (O_2/suction/air) as appropriate;

    - education (for whom?);

- traffic patterns for patients, health care staff and visitors.

- transport and disposal and route for waste.

- cleaning schedules for dust/debris control:

    - during;

    - in the event of incidence;

    - post construction/completion;

- infection control rounds/meetings with contractor;

- patient assessment – who is at risk?;

- any other controls necessary.

This must be agreed and signed by all parties prior to commencement of work.

2. Involvement in initial planning and approval meetings at design stage of project:

- number and type of hand wash basins and complete system (soap, towels, alcohol dispenser, waste bins);

- number and type of single rooms/bays;

- heating, temperature-control, ventilation and grilles;

- plumbing, radiators, inspection hatches;

- number and fixings for sharps dispensers;

- fixtures and fittings – ease of cleaning;

- surfaces – ceilings, walls, worktops, floors;

- ancillary rooms – DU, CU, disposal hold, washing facilities etc;

- type of storage facilities.

3. Ensure major design components in place to support infection control practice (see Chapter 4).

4. Ensure preparation for demolition and construction are complete and all parties understand the importance of compliance with the policies concerned, that is, contractors, managers, healthcare staff and patients.

5. Environmental rounds should check:

- dust, debris control;

- traffic control;

- barrier systems in place if appropriate;

- cleanliness of any adjoining areas plus site;

- air flow;

- temperature/humidity;

- contamination of patient rooms, supplies and equipment.

6. Check post-construction clean-up:

- contractors;

- domestic;

- estates.

7. Check design to support infection control practice has been achieved. See Bartley (2000) for further guidance.

8. Providing a built environment that promotes good infection control depends on the following factors:

- ascertaining who is to responsible for infection control needs;

- establishing specific goals of infection control in relation to the function of the facilities to be built or refurbished;

- agreeing the agenda for achieving "designed-in" infection control;

- planning the built environment in relation to infection control considerations;

- implementing the programme and co-ordinating the involvement of the infection control team;

- improving communication between professionals in the health facilities management and building sectors;

- disseminating findings related to best practice in design for good infection control and promoting economies of scale by replicating good infection control design components where possible;

- improving the information base for building industry professionals and infection control teams;

- monitoring new developments based on research.

9. Common pitfalls arise from a number of pressures, for example the pressure to choose the cheapest design or product. As many authors have argued, the best designs or products may be more expensive initially but in the long term they will inevitably realise cost benefits as they may prevent outbreaks, last longer, require less maintenance and be more durable and easier to clean.

Appendix 7 Glossary

Airborne infection: A mechanism of transmission of an infectious agent by particles, dust, or droplet nuclei suspended in the air (Last, 1995).

Aspergillosis: A fungal infection caused by *Aspergillus* spp., commonly found in soil, decaying vegetable matter, damp cellars, building materials and ventilation systems. The most common mode of transmission is by the airborne route, for example dispersal of a contaminated aerosol. In fact, airborne aspergillosis is a risk to patients with highly compromised immunity.

Contact transmission has been reported, for example a recent cluster of cases in Manchester suggested a contaminated stockinette was the source of infection. The density of *Aspergillus* spp. spores in hospital air is increased considerably during construction, and there is evidence that healthcare-associated aspergillosis is caused by contamination of ward air from outside. Hospital ventilation systems can draw in contaminated outside air because of either malfunction or inadequate mechanical ventilation and air filtration (Manuel and Kibbler, 1998; Cornet et al, 1999; Mahieu et al, 2000; Richardson et al, 2000; Thio et al, 2000).

At-risk patient: Susceptible patient: a patient with considerably reduced immunological competence who has a pre-existing pathology that may compromise their immune status (for example cancer, diabetes, chronic cirrhosis, hypoparathyroidism), or who is subjected to extensive invasive procedures (Worsley et al, 1990; Manuel and Kibbler, 1998). The vulnerability of a patient in relation to developing an infectious disease after contact with any given causal agent is governed by a number of factors. These include the virulence and dose of the infectious agent, previous exposure to the organism or an antigenic component, for example vaccination, age of the individual, nutritional state of the person, the presence of other diseases and whether the individual is receiving immunosuppressive therapy (Donaldson and Donaldson, 2000).

Bandolier: A print and Internet journal about healthcare, using evidence-based medicine techniques to provide advice about particular treatments or diseases for healthcare professionals and consumers.

Bay: see **Single room**

Clinical governance: A framework through which NHS organisations are accountable for continuously improving the quality of their services, safeguarding high standards by creating an environment in which excellence in clinical care will flourish ('A First class service', Department of Health).

Cohort barrier nursing: see **Cohorting**

Cohorting: Placing patients infected with the same micro-organism (but with no other infection) in a discrete clinical area where they are cared for by staff who are restricted to these patients.

Communicable disease: (synonym = infectious disease) An illness due to a specific infectious agent or its toxic products that arises through transmission of that agent or its products from an infected person, animal, or reservoir to a susceptible host, either directly or indirectly through an intermediate plant or animal host, vector, or the inanimate environment.

Contact: Association with an infected person or animal or a contaminated environment such that there is an opportunity to acquire the infection.

Contamination: The presence of an infectious agent on a body surface; also on or in clothes, bedding, toys, surgical instruments or dressings, or other inanimate articles or substances including water and food. Contamination does not imply a carrier state.

Cross-infection: An infection either due to a microbe that came from another patient, member of staff or visitor in a healthcare establishment or due to a microbe that originated in the inanimate environment of the patient.

Dead-legs: In a water supply and distribution system, pipes that are capped off or rarely used.

Direct contact: Refers to a mode of transmission of infection between an infected host and a susceptible host. Direct contact occurs when skin or mucous surfaces touch, for example hand contact.

En-suite single room: see **Single room**

Fomites: Articles that convey infection to others because they have been contaminated by pathogenic organisms. Examples include hospital equipment, instruments, kidney dishes, hospital bed tables, drinking glasses, door handles, clothing and toys (Last, 1995).

Fungi: Unicellular, multicellular or syncytial spore-forming organisms that feed on organic matter; includes yeasts and moulds (Baril, 2000). The most common fungal infections are caused by *Candida* spp. (see, for example, O'Connell and Humphreys, 2000).

Gram-negative bacteria: Group of bacteria that (after a staining procedure) stain red when viewed under the microscope. This group includes *Escherichia coli*, *Pseudomonas* spp. and *Shigella* spp. They are the main strains of bacteria in healthcare-associated infections.

Gram-positive bacteria: Group of bacteria that stain blue when viewed under a microscope. This group includes *Staphylococcus* spp. and *Streptococcus* spp.

Healthcare-associated infections: Infections that a patient acquires during a visit to, or that is related to a stay in, a healthcare facility.

Heat labile: That which is likely to be damaged or destroyed by the normal heat disinfection process.

Iatrogenic infection: Infection that arises as an unwanted consequence of a medical intervention.

Immunocompromised patient: A patient whose immune response is deficient because of an impaired immune system. See also **At-risk patient**.

Indirect contact: A mode of transmission of infection involving fomites or vectors. Vectors may be mechanical or biological.

Isolation room: see **Single room**

Mode of transmission: see **Transmission**

Non-touch (taps): Includes foot- or knee-operated, or infrared sensor taps.

Pathogen: A bacterium, virus, or other micro-organism that can cause disease.

Prion: An infectious protein, to which several so-called slow virus diseases (for example Creutzfeldt–Jakob Disease, scrapie, and bovine spongiform encephalopathy) are attributed. The word was coined in 1982 by S. Prusiner, from *proteinaceous infectious* particles, reversing the order of the vowels.

Reservoir (of infection): Any person, animal, plant, soil, or substance, or a combination of these, in which an infectious agent normally lives and multiplies, on which it depends primarily for survival, and where it reproduces itself in such a manner that it can be transmitted to a susceptible host: the natural habitat of the infectious agent (Last, 1995; Dancer, 1999).

Scale: a ratio representing the relationship between a specified distance on a sketch plan and the actual distance on the ground. For example, at the scale of 1:50, 1 unit of measurement on the plan equals 50 units of the same measurement on the ground.

Single room/En-suite single room/Isolation room/Bay: For the purposes of this document, the following terminology is used:

(1) **Single room:** This is a room with space for one patient and usually contains as a minimum: a bed; locker/wardrobe; and clinical hand-wash basin plus a small cupboard with worktop.

(2) **En-suite single room** – as above but with any combination of en-suite facility, i.e. shower, shower and toilet, bath and toilet or just toilet, etc.

(3) **Isolation room** – as in 1 and 2 but with either negative pressure ventilation for infectious patients (source isolation) or positive pressure for immunocompromised patients (protective isolation). May or may not have a lobby or en-suite facility.

(4) **Bay** is any room that contains more than one bed (i.e. two-bedded bay; three-bedded bay; four-bedded bay; six-bedded bay, etc.) which may or may not have en-suite facilities.

Spore: Some species of bacteria, particularly those of the genera *Bacillus* and *Clostridium*, which are significant cause of infection in humans, develop highly resistant structures called spores when they are exposed to adverse conditions, such as a lack of nutrients or water. Spores are resistant to disinfectants and to high or low temperatures. They may remain viable for many years but when the environment conditions improve the spores germinate and the bacterial cell inside starts to multiply again.

Thermostatic mixing valves: Valves that mix the hot and cold water of the system to provide water at a predetermined temperature.

Transmissible Spongiform Encephalopathy (TSE): Name for a group of fatal degenerative brain diseases that causes sponge-like abnormalities in brain cells. TSE diseases are associated with accumulation of abnormal prion protein in the brain.

Transmission: Any mechanism by which an infectious agent is spread from a source or reservoir to a person. Modes of transmission of infection include direct transmission involving direct transfer of micro-organisms to the skin or mucous membranes by direct contact; indirect transmission involves an intermediate stage between the source of infection and the individual, for example infected food, water or vector-borne transmission by insects; airborne transmission involving inhaling aerosols containing micro-organisms, for example legionnaires' disease or tuberculosis (Last, 1995; Donaldson and Donaldson, 2000).

References

ACTS AND REGULATIONS

Construction (Design and Management) Regulations 1994, SI 1994 No. 3140, The Stationery Office.
http://www.hmso.gov.uk/si/si1994/Uksi_19943140_en_1.htm

Construction (Design and Management) (Amendment) Regulations 2000, SI 2000 No 2380, The Stationery Office.
http://www.legislation.hmso.gov.uk/si/si2000/20002380.htm

Control of Substances Hazardous to Health (COSHH) Regulations 1999, SI 1999 No. 437, The Stationery Office.
http://www.hmso.gov.uk/si/si1999/19990437.htm

Environmental Protection Act 1990, The Stationery Office.
http://www.hmso.gov.uk/acts/acts1990/Ukpga_19900043_en_1.htm

Food Safety Act 1990, The Stationery Office.
http://www.hmso.gov.uk/acts/acts1990/Ukpga_19900016_en_1.htm

Health and Safety at Work etc Act 1974, The Stationery Office.

Water Supply (Water Fittings) Regulations 1999, SI 1999 No. 1148, The Stationery Office.
http://www.legislation.hmso.gov.uk/si/si1999/19991148.htm

Water Supply (Water Fittings) (Amendment) Regulations 1999, SI 1999 No. 1506, The Stationery Office.
http://www.legislation.hmso.gov.uk/si/si1999/19991506.htm

Water Supply (Water Quality) Regulations 2000, SI 2000 No. 3184, The Stationery Office.
http://www.hmso.gov.uk/si/si2000/20003184.htm

Water Supply (Water Quality) (Amendment) Regulations 2001, SI 2001 No. 2885, The Stationery Office.
http://www.legislation.hmso.gov.uk/si/si2001/20012885.htm

Workplace (Health, Safety and Welfare) Regulations 1992, SI 1992 No.3004, The Stationery Office.
http://www.hmso.gov.uk/si/si1992/Uksi_19923004_en_1.htm

BRITISH STANDARDS

BS 6920 – Part 1:2000 Suitability of non-metallic products for use in contact with water intended for human consumption with regard to their effect on the quality of water

BS EN 12056: Gravity drainage systems inside buildings.

Part 1:2000　General and performance requirements.

Part 2:2000　Sanitary pipework, layout and calculation.

Part 3:2000　Roof drainage, layout and calculation.

Part 4:2000　Wastewater lifting plants. Layout and calculation.

Part 5:2000　Installation and testing, instructions for operation, maintenance and use.

NHS ESTATES

[NOTE: As guidance documents are being constantly updated, it is advisable that readers check the NHS Estates website for the most up-to-date publications list and the latest information on the more recent revisions: http://www.nhsestates.gov.uk/publications_guidance/index.asp]

Health Building Notes

HBN 4: In-patient accommodation – options for choice, HMSO, 1997.

HBN 6: Facilities for diagnostic imaging and interventional radiology, The Stationery Office, London, 2001.

HBN 8: Facilities for rehabilitation services, HMSO, 2000.

HBN 10: Catering department, HMSO, 1997.

HBN 12: Out-patient department, HMSO, 1990.

HBN 13: Sterile services department, HMSO, 1993.

HBN 15: Accommodation for pathology services, HMSO, 1991.

HBN 25: Laundry, HMSO, 1994.

HBN 26: Operating department, HMSO, 1991.

HBN 36 Vol 1 – Local healthcare facilities, HMSO, 1995.

HBN 52: Accommodation for day care:

Vol. 1 – day surgery unit, HMSO, 1993.

Vol. 2 – endoscopy unit, HMSO, 1994.

Vol. 3 – medical investigation and treatment unit, HMSO, 1995.

HBN 57: Critical care facilities, The Stationery Office, London, 2002.

Health Technical Memoranda

HTM 55: Windows, HMSO, 1998.

HTM 56: Partitions, HMSO, 1998.

HTM 58: Internal doorsets, HMSO, 1998.

HTM 60: Ceilings, HMSO, 1989.

HTM 61: Flooring, HMSO, 1995.

HTM 64: Sanitary assemblies, HMSO, 1995.

HTM 2007: Electrical services: supply and distribution:

Management policy, HMSO, 1993.

Design considerations, HMSO, 1993.

Validation and verification, HMSO, 1993.

Operational management, HMSO, 1993.

HTM 2009: Pneumatic air tube transport systems:

Management policy, HMSO, 1995.

Design considerations and Good practice guide, HMSO, 1995.

HTM 2010: Sterilization:

Management policy, HMSO, 1994.

Design considerations, HMSO, 1995.

Validation and verification, HMSO, 1995.

Good practice guide, HMSO, 1995.

Operational management with testing and validation protocols, HMSO, 1997.

HTM 2022: Medical gas pipeline systems

Design, installation, validation and verification, HMSO, 1997.

Operational management, HMSO, 1997.

HTM 2025: Ventilation in healthcare premises:

Management policy, HMSO, 1994.

Design considerations, HMSO, 1994.

Validation and verification, HMSO, 1994.

Operational management, HMSO, 1994.

HTM 2027: Hot and cold water supply, storage and mains services:

Management policy, HMSO, 1995.

Design considerations, HMSO, 1995.

Operational management, HMSO, 1995.

Validation and verification, HMSO, 1995.

HTM 2030: Washer-disinfectors:

Design considerations, HMSO, 1997.

HTM 2040: Control of legionellae in healthcare premises – A code of practice:

Design considerations, HMSO, 1994.

HTM 2065: Healthcare waste management – segregation of waste streams in clinical areas, HMSO, 1997.

Health Guidance Notes

Safe disposal of clinical waste: whole hospital policy guidance, HMSO, 1995.

Other NHS Estates publications

Housekeeping: a first guide to new, modern and dependable ward housekeeping services in the NHS, The Stationery Office, 2001.
http://www.nhsestates.gov.uk/download/publications_guidance/housekeeping.pdf

National standards of cleanliness for the NHS, The Stationery Office, 2001.
http://www.nhsestates.gov.uk/download/cleaning_standards/NHS_cleaning_standards.pdf

Ward layouts with privacy and dignity, The Stationery Office, forthcoming (see NHS Estates website for updates).

DEPARTMENT OF HEALTH

Health Service Circulars

http://www.doh.gov.uk/coinh.htm

'Decontamination of medical devices', HSC 2000/032.

'The management and control of hospital infection', HSC 2000/002.

'Governance in the new NHS: controls assurance statements 1999/2000 – risk management and organisational controls', HSC 1999/123.

'Resistance to antibiotics and other antimicrobial agents', HSC 1999/049.

Health Service Guidelines

'Management of food hygiene and food services in the NHS', HSG(96)20.
http://tap.ccta.gov.uk/doh/coin4.nsf/page/HSG-(96)20?OpenDocument

'Hospital infection control', HSG(95)10, 1995.

'Hospital laundry arrangements for used and infected linen', HSG(95)18, 1995.

Other DoH publications

Advisory Committee on Dangerous Pathogens: **Protection against blood-borne infections in the workplace: HIV and Hepatitis**, HMSO, 1995.
http://www.doh.gov.uk/bbinf.htm

A protocol for the local decontamination of surgical instruments, 2001.
http://www.doh.gov.uk/decontaminationguidance/decon.pdf

Assured safe catering – a management system for hazard analysis, The Stationery Office, 1993.

Controls Assurance Standard: Infection Control, Rev 02(2001). http://www.doh.gov.uk/riskman.htm

Decontamination Programme Technical Manual – Part 1: Process Assessment Tool and Decontamination Guidance (updated), 2001.
http://www.nhsestates.gov.uk/facilities_management/index.asp?submenu_ID=decontamination

Decontamination Programme Technical Manual – Part 2: Decontamination Organisational Review Information System (DORIS).
http://www.nhsestates.gov.uk/facilities_management/index.asp?submenu_ID=decontamination

A First Class Service, HMSO, 1998.

Hospital catering: delivering a quality service, 1996.

NHS Plan Implementation Programme, 2000.
http://www.doh.gov.uk/nhsplanimpprogramme

Public-Private Partnerships in the National Health Service: The Private Finance Initiative, HMSO, 1999.

Risk assessment for transmission of vCJD via surgical instruments: a modelling approach and numerical scenarios, Economics and Operational Research Division, 2001.
http://www.doh.gov.uk/cjd/riskassessmentsi.htm

The NHS Plan (2000).
http://www.nhs.uk/nationalplan/

The operating room of the year 2010: a report to the Department of Trade and Industry, 1999.
http://tap.ccta.gov.uk/doh/point.nsf/page/CC8668247645AA1A002567060045D1C2?OpenDocument

The path of least resistance, Standing Medical Advisory Committee Sub-Group on Antimicrobial Resistance, 1998.
http://www.doh.gov.uk/smac1.htm

UK antimicrobial resistance strategy and action plan, 2000.
http://www.doh.gov.uk/arbstrat.htm

OTHER PUBLICATIONS (INCLUDING EVIDENCE-BASED RESEARCH)

Alberti, C, Bouakline, A, Ribaud, P, Lacroix, C, Rousselot, P, Leblanc, T and Derouin, F (2001), *Relationship between environmental fungal contamination and the incidence of invasive aspergillosis in haematology patients*, **Journal of Hospital Infection**, Vol 48 No 3, July, pp 198–206.
http://www.harcourt-international.com/journals/jhin/previous.cfm?art=jhin.2001.0998

Archibald, LK, Manning, ML, Bell, LM, Banerjee, S and Jarvis, WR (1997), *Patient density, nurse-to-patient ratio and nosocomial infection risk in a pediatric cardiac intensive care unit*, **Pediatric Infectious Disease Journal**, Vol 16 No 11, November, pp 1045–1050.
http://www.lww.com/PIDJ/0891-366811-97toc.html

Audit Commission (1997), **Getting sorted: the safe and economic management of hospital waste**, Audit Commission Publications, ISBN 1-86240-017-2.
http://www.audit-commission.gov.uk/ac2/NR/Health/ebnh0397.htm

Ayliffe, GAJ, Collins, BJ and Taylor, LJ (1999), **Hospital-Acquired Infection: Principles and Prevention**, Butterworth-Heinemann, London.

Ayliffe, GAJ, Fraise, AP, Geddes, AM and Mitchell, K (2000), **Control of Infection: A Practical Handbook**, 4th edition, Chapman & Hall Medical, London.

Baril, G (2000), *Rx for SBS*, **Health Facilities Management**, April, p 26.

Barnett, J, Thomlinson, D, Perry, C, Marshall, R and MacGowan, AP (1999), *An audit of the use of manual handling equipment and their microbiological flora – implications for infection control*, **Journal of Hospital Infection**, Vol 43 No 4, pp 309–313.
http://www.harcourt-international.com/journals/jhin/previous.cfm?art=jhin.1999.0646

Barrie, D (1998), *Central Sterilising Club – Laundry Working Group*, Discussion Paper, **CSC Bulletin**, Vol 3 No 1.

Bartley, JM (2000), *APIC state-of-the-art report: the role of infection control during construction in health care facilities*, **American Journal of Infection Control** (AJIC), Vol 28 No 2, April, pp 156–169.

Bernard, L, Kereveur, A, Durand, D, Gonot, J, Goldstein, F, Mainardi, JL, Acar, J and Carlet, J (1999), *Bacterial contamination of hospital physicians' stethoscopes*, **Infection Control and Hospital Epidemiology**, Vol 20 No 9, September, pp 626–628.
http://www.slackinc.com/general/iche/stor0999/9car.htm

Blackmore, M (1987), *Hand-drying methods*, **Nursing Times**, Vol 83 No 37, pp 71–74.

Blenkharn, JI (1995), *The disposal of clinical waste*, **Journal of Hospital Infection**, Vol 30 supplement, June, pp 514–520.

Bonten, MJ, Hayden, MK, Nathan, C, van Voorhis, J, Matushek, M, Slaughter, S, Rice, T and Weinstein, RA (1996), *Epidemiology of colonisation of patients and environment with vancomycin-resistant enterococci*, **Lancet**, Vol 348 No 9042, 14 December, pp 1615–1619.

Bosshammer, J, Fiedler, B, Gudowius, P, von der Hardt, H, Romling, U and Tummler, B (1995), *Comparative hygienic surveillance of contamination with pseudomonas in a cystic fibrosis ward over a 4 year period*, **Journal of Hospital Infection**, Vol 31 No 4, December, pp 261–274.

Boyce, J, Kelliher, S and Vallande, N (2000), *Skin irritation and dryness associated with two hand-hygiene regimens: soap-and-water hand washing versus hand antisepsis with an alcoholic hand gel*, **Infection Control and Hospital Epidemiology**, Vol 21 No 7, July, pp 443–448.
http://www.slackinc.com/general/iche/stor0700/7boy.htm

Boyce, JM, Potter-Bynoe, G, Chenevert, C and King, T (1997), *Environmental contamination due to MRSA: possible infection control implications*, **Infection Control and Hospital Epidemiology**, Vol 18 No 9, September, pp 622–627.
http://www.slackinc.com/general/iche/stor0997/boyce.htm

Burnett, IA, Weeks, GR and Harris, DM (1994), *A hospital study of ice making machines: their bacteriology design, usage and upkeep*, **Journal of Hospital Infection**, Vol 28 No 4, pp 305–313.

Burns, DN, Wallace, RJ Jr, Schultz, ME, Zhang, YS, Zubairi, SQ, Pang, YJ, Gibert, CL, Brown, BA, Noel, ES and Gordin, FM (1991), *Nosocomial outbreak of respiratory tract colonization with* Mycobacterium fortuitum: *demonstration of the usefulness of pulsed-field gel electrophoresis in an epidemiologic investigation*, **American Review of Respiratory Disease**, Vol 144 No 5, November, pp 1153–1159.

Bushell, J (2000), "In design of new and refurbished buildings", in McCulloch, J (Ed), **Infection Control: Science, Management and Practice**, Whurr, London (Chapter 5).

Carter, C and Barr, B (1997), *Infection control issues in construction and renovation*, **Infection Control and Hospital Epidemiology**, Vol 18 No 8, August, pp 587–596.

Cartmill, TDI, Panigrahi, H, Worsley, MA, McCann, DC, Nice, CN and Keith, E (1994), *Management and control of a large outbreak of diarrhoea due to* Clostridium difficile, **Journal of Hospital Infection**, Vol 27, pp 1–15.

CDC (1994), *Guidelines for preventing the transmission of Mycobacterium tuberculosis in health care facilities*, US Department of Health and Human Services, Public Health Service, MMWR 43(RR13).
http://wonder.cdc.gov/wonder/prevguid/m0035909/m0035909.asp

CDC (1995), *Recommendations for preventing the spread of vancomycin resistance: recommendations of the Hospital Infection Control Practices Advisory Committee (HICPAC)*, **MMWR Morbidity and Mortality Weekly Report**, 44(RR-12), pp 1–13.
http://aepo-xdv-www.epo.cdc.gov/wonder/prevguid/m0039349/m0039349.asp

CDC (1997), **Guidelines for isolation precautions in hospitals. Part II. Recommendations for isolation precautions in hospitals**, Hospital Infection Control Practices Advisory Committee
http://www.cdc.gov/ncidod/hip/isolat/isopart2.htm

Chadwick, PR, Beards, G, Brown, D, Caul, EO, Cheesebrough, J, Clarke, I, Curry, A, O'Brien, S, Quigley, K, Sellwood, J and Westmoreland, D (2000), *Management of hospital outbreaks of gastro-enteritis due to small round structured viruses (Report of the Public Health Laboratory Service Viral Gastro-enteritis Working Group)*, **Journal of Hospital Infection**, Vol 45, May, pp 1–10.
http://www.harcourt-international.com/journals/jhin/previous.cfm?art=jhin.2000.0662

Chartered Institution of Building Services Engineers (1999), **CIBSE Guide Vol. G: Public health engineering**, 222 Balham High Road, Balham, London SW12 9BS.

Cheesbrough, JS, Barkess-Jones, L and Brown, DW (1997), *Possible prolonged environmental survival of small, round structured viruses*, **Journal of Hospital Infection**, Vol 35 No 4, April, pp 325–326.

Claesson, BE and Claesson, UL (1995), *An outbreak of endometritis in a maternity unit caused by spread of Group streptococci from a shower head*, **Journal of Hospital Infection**, Vol 6 No 3, pp 304–311.

Collins, BJ (1988), *The hospital environment; how clean should a hospital be?*, **Journal of Hospital Infection**, Vol 11, Supplement A, February, pp 53–56.

Commons Public Accounts Committee (2000), **Forty-second Report: The Management and Control of Hospital Acquired Infection in Acute NHS Trusts in England**, 23 November, London, HC 620 ISBN 0-10-269500-8.

Cornet, M, Levy, V, Fleury, L, Lortholary, J, Barquins, S, Coureul, M-H, Deliere, E, Zittoun, R, Brücker, G and Bouvet, A (1999), *Efficacy of prevention by high-efficiency particulate air filtration or laminar airflow against Aspergillus airborne contamination during hospital renovation*, **Infection Control and Hospital Epidemiology**, Vol 20 No 7, pp 508–513.
http://www.slackinc.com/general/iche/stor0799/cor.htm

Cotterill, S, Evans, R and Fraise, AP (1996), *An unusual source for an outbreak of methicillin-resistant Staphylococcus aureus on an intensive therapy unit*, **Journal of Hospital Infection**, Vol 32 No 3, March, pp 207–216.

Dan, BR (1980), *Bacteraemia tied to overcrowding, overtime and decreased hand washing*, **Hospital Infection Control**, Vol 7 No 6, June, pp 61–62.

Dancer, SJ (1999), *Mopping up hospital infection*, **Journal of Hospital Infection**, Vol 43 No 2, October, pp 85–100.
http://www.harcourt-international.com/journals/jhin/previous.cfm?art=jhin.1999.0616

Dennis, G, Maki, MD, Carla, J, Alvarado, BS, Carol, A, Hassemer, BS and Zilz, MA (1982), *Relation of the inanimate hospital environment to endemic nosocomial infection*, **New England Journal of Medicine**, Vol 307 No 25, 16 December, pp 1562–1566.

Dobson, C et al (1997), *Silver/copper ionisation treatment of water to reduce the risk of Legionella in NHS healthcare premises*, **Health Estate Journal**, May, pp 7–10.

Duckworth, GJ and Jordens, JZ (1990), *Adherence and survival properties of an epidemic methicillin resistant strain of Staphylococcus aureus compared with those of methicillin sensitive strains*, **Journal of Medical Microbiology**, Vol 32, pp 195–200.

Feather, A, Stone, SP, Wessier, A, Boursicot, KA and Pratt, C (2000), *"Now please wash your hands": the handwashing behaviour of final MBBS candidates*, **Journal of Hospital Infection**, Vol 45 No 1, May, pp 62–64.
http://www.harcourt-international.com/journals/jhin/previous.cfm?art=jhin.1999.0705

Finn, L and Crook, S (1998), *Minor surgery in general practice – setting the standards*, **Journal of Public Health Medicine**, Vol 20 No 2, pp 169–174.
http://www3.oup.co.uk:80/pubmed/hdb/Volume_20/Issue_02/200169.sgm.abs.html

Flynn, PM, Williams, BG, Hetherington, SV, Williams, BF, Fiannini, MA and Pearson, TA (1993), *Aspergillus terreus during hospital renovation*, **Journal of Hospital Infection and Hospital Epidemiology**, Vol 14 No 7, July, pp 363–365.

Fox, N (1997), *Space, sterility and surgery: circuits of hygiene in the operating theatre*, **Social Science & Medicine**, Vol 45 No 5, pp 649–657.
http://www.healthabstractsonline.com/healthab/show/Products/HAO/ssm_frame.htt

Gould, D (1994), *Making sense of hand hygiene*, **Nursing Times**, Vol 90 No 30, pp 63–64.

Gould, D (1997), *Hygenic hand decontamination*, **Journal of Wound Care**, Vol 6 No 2, Supplement, pp 1–13.

Graman, PS, Quinlan, GA and Rank, JA (1997), *Nosocomial Legionellosis traced to a contaminated ice machine*, **Infection Control and Epidemiology**, Vol 18 No 9, September, pp 637–640.
http://www.slackinc.com/general/iche/stor0997/gram.htm

Green, J, Right, PA, Gallimore, CI, Mitchell, O, Morgan-Capner, P and Brown, DWG (1998), *The role of environmental contamination with small round structured*

viruses in a hospital outbreak investigated by reverse-transcriptase polymerase chain reaction assay, **Journal of Hospital Infection**, Vol 39 No 1, May, pp 39–45.
http://www.harcourt-international.com/journals/jhin/previous.cfm?art=hi970363

Griffith, CJ, Cooper, RA, Gilmore, J, Davies, C and Lewis, M (2000), An evaluation of hospital cleaning regimes and standards, **Journal of Hospital Infection**, Vol 45 No 1, pp 19–28.
http://www.harcourt-international.com/journals/jhin/previous.cfm?art=jhin.1999.0717

Haley, RW and Bregman, DA (1982), The role of under staffing, over crowding in recurrent outbreaks of Staphylococcal infection in a neo-natal special care unit, **Journal of Infectious Diseases**, Vol 145 No 6, June, pp 875–885.

Hannan, MM, Azadian, BS, Gazzard, BG, Hawkins, DA and Hoffman, PN (2000), Hospital infection control in an era of HIV infection and multi-drug resistant tuberculosis, **Journal of Hospital Infection**, Vol 44 No 1, January, pp 5–11.
http://www.harcourt-international.com/journals/jhin/previous.cfm?art=jhin.1999.0651

Harris, AD, Samore, MH, Nafziger, R, DiRosario, K, Roghmann, MC and Carmeli, Y (2000), A survey on handwashing practices and opinions of healthcare workers, **Journal of Hospital Infection**, Vol 45 No 4, August, pp 318–321.
http://www.harcourt-international.com/journals/jhin/previous.cfm?art=jhin.2000.0781

Health & Safety Commission (2001), **Legionnaires' disease: the control of legionella bacteria in water systems – Approved Code of Practice and Guidance**, ISBN 0-7176-1772-6, HSE Books, Suffolk.
http://www.hsebooks.co.uk/

Health and Safety Executive (1999), 'Safe use of pneumatic air tube transport systems for pathology specimens', HSE Information Sheet, MISC 186.
http://www.hse.gov.uk/pubns/misc186.pdf

Health Services Advisory Committee and the Environment Agency (1999), **Safe Disposal of Clinical Waste**, ISBN 0-7176-2492-7, HSE Books.

Hill, AF, Butterworth, RJ, Joiner, S, Jackson, G, Rossor, MN, Thomas, DJ, Frosh, A, Tolley, N, Bell, JE, Spencer, M, King, A, Al-Sarraj, S, Ironside, JW, Lantos, PL and Collinge, J (1999), Investigation of variant Creutzfeldt–Jakob Disease and other human prion diseases with tonsil biopsy samples, **Lancet**, Vol 353, pp 183–189.

Hilton, DA, Fathers, E, Edwards, P, Ironside, JW and Zajicek, J (1998), Prion immunoreactivity in appendix before clinical onset of variant Creutzfeldt–Jakob disease, **Lancet**, Vol 352, pp 703–704.

Hirai, Y (1991), Survival of bacteria under dry conditions from a viewpoint of nosocomial infection, **Journal of Hospital Infection**, Vol 19 No 3, November, pp 191–200.

Hoffman, PN and Wilson, J (1994), Hands, hygiene and hospitals, **PHLS Microbiology Digest**, Vol 11 No 4, pp 211–261.

Hoffman, PN, Bennett, AM and Scott, GM (1999), Controlling airborne infections, **Journal of Hospital Infection**, Vol 43 (Supplement), pp S203–210.

Holton, J and Ridgway, GL (1993), Commissioning operating theatres, **Journal of Hospital Infection**, Vol 23, pp 161–167.

Hooper, DM (1994), One hospital's road to waste minimisation, **Medical Waste Analyst**, Vol 2 No 8, May, pp 1, 3–5.

Humphreys, H (1993), Infection control and the design of a new operating suite, **Journal of Hospital Infection**, Vol 23 No 1, pp 61–70.

Hunter, PR and Burge, SH (1988), Monitoring the bacteriological quality of potable waters in hospital, **Journal of Hospital Infection**, Vol 12, pp 289–294.

ICNA/ADM (1999), Standards Working Group. **Standards for environmental cleanliness in hospitals.**
http://www.icna.co.uk

Irwin, RS, Demers, RR, Pratter, MR et al (1980), An outbreak of Acinetobacter infection associated with the use of a ventilator spirometer, **Respiratory Care**, Vol 25, pp 232–237.

Kaplan, JE, Gary, BW, Baron, RC et al (1982), Epidemiology of Norwalk gastroenteritis and the role of Norwalk virus in outbreaks of acute non-bacterial gastroenteritis, **Annals of International Medicine**, Vol 96, pp 756–761.

Karanfil, LV, Murphy, M, Josephson, A, Gaynes, R, Mandel, L, Hill, BC and Swenson, JM (1992), A cluster of vancomycin-resistant enterococcus faecium in an intensive care unit, **Infection Control Hospital Epidemiology**, Vol 13 No 4, April, pp 195–200.

Kesavan, S, Barodowal, S and Mulley, GP (1998), Now wash your hands: a survey of hospital handwashing facilities, **Journal of Hospital Infection**, Vol 40 No 4, December, pp 291–293.
http://www.harcourt-international.com/journals/jhin/previous.cfm?art=hi980462

Keys, A, Baldwin, A and Austin, S (2000), *Reducing waste by design*, **Building Services Journal**, December, pp 49–50.

Kibbler, CC, Quick, A and O'Neill, AM (1998), *The effect of increased bed numbers on MRSA transmission in acute medical wards*, **Journal of Hospital Infection**, Vol 39 No 3, July, pp 213–219.
http://www.harcourt-international.com/journals/jhin/previous.cfm?art=hi970354

Kumari, DN, Haji, TC, Keer, V, Hawkey, PM, Duncanson, V and Flower, E (1998), *Ventilation grilles as a potential source of methicillin-resistant* Staphylococcus aureus *causing an outbreak in an orthopaedic ward at a district general hospital*, **Journal of Hospital Infection**, Vol 39 No 2, June, pp 127–133.
http://www.harcourt-international.com/journals/jhin/previous.cfm?art=hi980357

Lacey, RW, Barr, KW and Inglis, TJ (1986), *Properties of methicillin-resistant* Staphylococcus aureus *colonising patients in burns units*, **Journal of Hospital Infection**, Vol 7, pp 137–148.

Lambert, I, Tebbs, SE, Hill, D, Moss, HA, Davies, AJ and Elliott, TSJ (2000), *Interferential therapy machines as possible vehicles for cross-infection*, **Journal of Hospital Infection**, Vol 44 No 1, January, pp 59–64.
http://www.harcourt-international.com/journals/jhin/previous.cfm?art=jhin.1999.0647

Langley, JM, Hanakowski, M and Bortolussi, R (1994), *Demand for isolation beds in a paediatric hospital*, **American Journal of Infection Control**, Vol 22 No 4, pp 207–211.

Larson, E and Killien, M (1982), *Factors influencing hand washing behaviour of patient care personnel*, **American Journal of Infection Control**, Vol 10, pp 93–99.

Last, J (Ed) (1995), **A Dictionary of Epidemiology**, 3rd edition, Oxford University Press, New York.

Lidwell, OM, Lowbury, EJL, Whyte, W, Blowers, R, Stanley, ST and Lowe, D (1982), *Effect of ultra-clean air in operating theatres on deep sepsis in the joint after total hip or knee replacement: a randomised study*, **British Medical Journal**, Vol 285, pp 10–14.

Louther, J, Rivera, P, Feldman, J, Villa, R, DeHovitz, J and Sepkowitz, KA (1997), *Risk of tuberculin conversion according to occupation among health care workers at a New York city hospital*, **American Journal of Respiratory and Critical Medicine**, Vol 156, pp 201–205.

McCulloch, J (Ed) (2000), **Infection Control: Science, Management and Practice**, Whurr, London.

Mahieu, L, De Dooy, JJ, Van Laer, FA, Jansens, H and Ieven, MM (2000), *A prospective study on factors influencing aspergillus spore load in the air during renovation works in a neonatal intensive care unit*, **Journal of Hospital Infection**, Vol 45 No 3, July, pp 191–197.
http://www.harcourt-international.com/journals/jhin/previous.cfm?art=jhin.2000.0773

Mallison, GF and Hayley, RW (1981), *Microbiological sampling of the inanimate environment in US hospitals 1976–1977*, **American Journal of Medicine**, Vol 70, pp 941–946.

Manangan, LP, Anderson, RL, Arduino, MJ and Bond, WW (1998), *Sanitary care and maintenance of ice storage chests and ice making machines in health care facilities*, **American Journal of Infection Control**, Vol 2, pp 111–112.
http://www.apic.org/ajic/

Manuel, R and Kibbler, C (1998), *The epidemiology and prevention of invasive aspergillosis*, **Journal of Hospital Infection**, Vol 39 No 2, June, pp 95–109.
http://www.harcourt-international.com/journals/jhin/previous.cfm?art=hi980365

Mermel, LA, Josephson, SL, Giorgio, CH, Dempsey, J and Parenteau, S (1995), *Association of legionnaires' disease with construction: contamination of potable water?*, **Journal of Infection Control and Hospital Epidemiology**, Vol 16 No 2, pp 76–81.

Microbiology Advisory Committee (1999), **Sterilisation, disinfection and cleaning of medical equipment: guidance on decontamination**, distributed by the Medical Devices Agency, February.
http://www.medical-devices.gov.uk/mda/mdawebsitev2.ns4/webvwOtherPublications/79735613F4BCC36100256ABD002F8AB5?OPEN

Miller, R and Swensson, E (1995), **New Directions in Hospitals and Healthcare Facility Design**, McGraw–Hill, New York, NY.

Miyamoto, M, Yamaguchi, Y and Sasatsu, M (2000), *Disinfectant effects of hot water, ultraviolet light, silver ions and chlorine on strains of Legionella and non-tuberculous mycobacteria*, **Microbios**, Vol 101 No 398, pp 7–13.

Moritz, JM (1995), *Current legislation governing clinical waste disposal*, **Journal of Hospital Infection**, Vol 30, Supplement, June, pp 521–530.

Musa, EK, Desai, N and Casewell, MW (1990), *The survival of* Acinetobacter calcoaceticus *inoculated on fingertips and on formica*, **Journal of Hospital Infection**, Vol 15 No 3, April, pp 219–227.

National Audit Office (2000), **Report by the Comptroller and Auditor General: The Management and Control of Hospital-acquired Infection in Acute NHS Trusts in England**, The Stationery Office, London.
http://www.nao.gov.uk/publications/nao_reports/9900230.pdf

Neely, AC and Maley, MP (2000), *Survival of enterococci and staphylococci on hospital fabrics and plastics*, **Journal of Clinical Microbiology**, Vol 38, pp 724–726.

Noskin, GA, Bednarz, P, Suriano, T, Reiner, S and Peterson, LR (2000), *Persistent contamination of fabric covered furniture by vancomycin-resistant enterococci: implications for upholstery selection in hospitals*, **American Journal of Hospital Infection**, Vol 22, pp 212–217.

O'Connell, NH and Humphreys, H (2000), *Intensive care unit design and environmental factors in the acquisition of infection*, **Journal of Hospital Infection**, Vol 45 No 4, August, pp 255–262.
http://www.harcourt-international.com/journals/jhin/previous.cfm?art=jhin.2000.0768

Palmer, R (1999), *Bacterial contamination of curtains in clinical areas*, **Nursing Standard**, Vol 14 No 2, 29 September–5 October, pp 33–35.

Phillips, G (1999), *Microbiological aspects of clinical waste*, **Journal of Hospital Infection**, Vol 41 No 1, January, pp 1–6.
http://www.harcourt-international.com/journals/jhin/previous.cfm?art=jhin.1998.0470

Picard, B and Goullet, P (1987), *Seasonal prevalence of nosocomial* Aeromonas hydrophila *infection related to aeromonas in hospital water*, **Journal of Hospital Infection**, Vol 10, pp 152–155.

Pittet, D (2000), *Improving compliance with hand hygiene in hospitals*, **Infection Control and Hospital Epidemiology**, Vol 21 No 6, pp 381–386.
http://www.slackinc.com/general/iche/stor0600/6pit.htm

Pittet, D, Hugonnet, S, Harbarth, S, Mourouga, P, Sauvan, V, Touveneau S et al (2000), *Effectiveness of a hospital-wide programme to improve compliance with hand hygiene*, **Lancet**, Vol 356, pp 1307–1312.

Plowman, R, Graves, N, Griffin, M, Roberts, JA, Swan, AV, Cookson, BD and Taylor, L (2000), **Socio-economic Burden of Hospital-acquired Infection**, Department of Health.
http://www.doh.gov.uk/haicosts.htm

Pratt, RJ, Pellowe, C, Loveday, HP, Robinson, N, Smith, GW and the EPIC Guideline Development Team (2000), *Phase I: Guidelines for preventing hospital-acquired infections*, **Journal of Hospital Infection**, Vol 47 (Supplement), S1–S42.

Rampling, A, Wiseman, S, Davis, L, Hyett, AP, Walbridge, A, Payne, G and Cornaby, AJ (2001), *Evidence that hospital hygiene is important in the control of methicillin-resistant* Staphylococcus aureus, **Journal of Hospital Infection**, Vol 49 No 2, October, pp 109–116.
http://www.harcourt-international.com/journals/jhin/previous.cfm?art=jhin.2001.1013

Richardson, MD, Rennie, S, Marshall, I, Morgan, MG, Murphy, JA, Shankland, GS, Watson, WH and Soutar, RL (2000), *Fungal surveillance of an open haematology ward*, **Journal of Hospital Infection**, Vol 45 No 4, August, pp 288–292.
http://www.harcourt-international.com/journals/jhin/previous.cfm?art=jhin.2000.0780

Rutala, WA and Weber, DJ (1999), *Infection control: the role of disinfection and sterilisation*, **Journal of Hospital Infection**, Vol 43 (Supplement), pp 843–855.

Saksena, NK, Song, JZ, Dwyer, DE and Cunningham, A (1999), 'Significance of simultaneous use of multiple HIV-1 genomic regions from cell-free and cell-associated virus in establishing epidemiologic linkage between 4 individuals who acquired HIV via surgical procedure', **6th Conference on Retrovirus and Opportunistic Infections**, Chicago, February.

Sanchez, RO and Hernandez, JM (1999), *Infection control during construction and renovation in the operating room*, **Seminars in Perioperative Nursing**, Vol 8 No 4, October, pp 208–214.

Sarangi, J and Roswell, R (1995), *Cleaning of carpets and soft furnishings*, **Journal of Hospital Infection**, Vol 30 No 2.

Sawyer, LA, Murphy, JJ and Kaplan, JE (1988), *25–30 mm virus particles associated with a hospital outbreak of acute gastroenteritis with evidence for airborne transmission*, **American Journal of Epidemiology**, Vol 127, pp 1261–1271.

Schaal, KP (1991), *Medical and microbiological problems arising from airborne infection in hospitals*, **Journal of Hospital Infection**, Vol 8 (Supplement A), pp 451–459.

Sherertz, RJ, Belani, A, Kramer, BS, Elfenbein, GJ, Weiner, RS, Sullivan, ML, Thomas, RG and Samsa, GP (1987), *Impact of air filtration on nosocomial Aspergillus infections. Unique risk of bone marrow transplant recipients*, **American Journal of Medicine**, Vol 83 No 4, October, pp 709–718
http://www4.ncbi.nlm.nih.gov/htbin-post/Entrez/query?db=m&form=6&uid=88046838&Dopt=r

Skoutelis, AT, Westenfelder, GO, Beckerdite, M and Phair, JP (1994), *Hospital carpeting and epidemiology of* Clostridium difficile, **American Journal of Infection Control**, Vol 22 No 4, August, pp 212–217.

Smith, SM, Eng, RHK and Padberg, FT Jr (1996), *Survival of nosocomial pathogenic bacteria at ambient temperatures*, **Journal of Medicine**, Vol 27 Nos 5 and 6, pp 293–302.

Smith, TL, Iwen, PC, Olson, SB and Rupp, MF (1998), *Environmental contamination with vancomycin-resistant enterococci in an outpatient setting*, **Infection Control Hospital Epidemiology**, Vol 19, pp 515–518.
http://www.slackinc.com/general/iche/stor0798/ccsmi.htm

Sniadack, DH, Ostroff, SM, Karlik, MA, Smithwick, RW, Schwartz, B, Sprauer, MA, Silcox, VA and Good, RC (1993), *A nosocomial pseudo-outbreak of* Mycobacterium xenopi *due to a contaminated potable water supply: lessons in prevention*, **Infection Control and Hospital Epidemiology**, Vol 14 No 11, November, pp 636–641.

Spencer, RC (1997), *Hospital/clinical waste: a control of infection officer's view*, **PHLS Microbiology Digest**, Vol 14, pp 163–165.

Stacey, A, Burden P, Croton C and Jones, E (1998), *Contamination of television sets by methicillin-resistant* Staphylococcus aureus *(MRSA)*, **Journal of Hospital Infection** (Letters to the Editor), Vol 39, pp 243–244.

Standaert, SM, Hutcheson, RH and Schaffner, W (1994), *Nosocomial transmission of Salmonella gastro-enteritis to laundry workers in a nursing home*, **Infection Control and Hospital Epidemiology**, Vol 15 No 1, January, pp 22–26.

Steinert, M, Ockert, G, Luck, C and Hacker, J (1998), *Regrowth of* Legionella pneumophila *in a heat disinfected plumbing system*, **Zentralblatt für Bakteriologie**, Vol 288 No 3, November, pp 331–342.

Suzuki, A et al (1984), *Bacterial contamination of floors and other surfaces in operating rooms: a five year survey*, **Journal of Hygiene**, Vol 93, pp 559–566.

Talon, D (1999), *The role of the hospital environment in the epidemiology of multi-resistant bacteria*, **Journal of Hospital Infection**, Vol 43 No 1, September, pp 13–17.
http://www.harcourt-international.com/journals/jhin/previous.cfm?art=jhin.1999.0613

Thio, CL, Smith, D, Merz, WG, Streifel, AJ, Bova, G, Gay, L, Miller, CB and Perl, TM (2000), *Refinements of environmental assessment during an outbreak investigation of invasive Aspergillus in a leukemia and bone marrow transport unit*, **Infection Control and Hospital Epidemiology**, Vol 21 No 1, January, pp 18–23.
http://www.slackinc.com/general/iche/stor0100/1thi.htm

Tobin, JOH, Beare, J, Dunnill, MS et al (1980), *Legionnaires' disease in a transplant unit: isolation of the causative agent from shower baths*, **Lancet**, Vol 2, pp 118–121.

Wagenvoort, JHT, Davies, BI, Westermann, EJA, Werink, TJ and Toenbreker, HM (1993), *MRSA from air-exhaust channels*, **Lancet**, Vol 341, pp 840–841.

Water Regulations Advisory Scheme (WRAS) (2001), **Water Fittings and Materials Directory**, Oakdale, Gwent.
http://www.wras.co.uk/publications/Directory.htm

Wearmouth, P (1999), 'Aspergillus infection – risks with demolition and building alterations'. Letters to Heads of Estates and Facilities, NHS Estates, November.

Webster, CA, Crowe, M, Humphreys, H and Towner, KJ (1998), *Surveillance of an adult intensive care unit for long-term persistence of a multi-resistant strain of* Acinetobacter baumannii, **European Journal of Clinical Microbiology and Infectious Diseases**, Vol 17 No 3, March, pp 171–176.
http://link.springer-ny.com/link/service/journals/10096/bibs/8017003/80170171.htm

Wiggam, SL and Hayward, AC (2000), *Hospitals in England are failing to follow guidance for tuberculosis infection control – results of a National Survey*, **Journal of Hospital Infection**, Vol 46 No 4, December, pp 257–262.

Wilson, IG, Hogg, GM and Barr, JG (1997), *Microbiological quality of ice in hospital and community*, **Journal of Hospital Infection**, Vol 36 No 3, July; pp 171–180.
http://www.harcourt-international.com/journals/jhin/previous.cfm?art=hi970234

Worsley, M et al (Eds) (1990), **Infection Control: Guidelines for Nursing Care**, Infection Control Nurses Association.

Zafar, AB, Gaydos, LA, Furlong, WB, Nguyen MH and Mennonna PA (1998), *Effectiveness of infection control programme in controlling nosocomial* Clostridium difficile, **American Journal of Infection Control**, Vol 26, pp 588–593.

FURTHER READING

Abrutyn, NE (Ed)(1998), **Infection Control Reference Service**. WB Saunders Co, Philadelphia, PA, ISBN 072-166-4431.

American Institute of Architects/Academy of Architecture for Health (1996), **Guidelines for design and construction of hospital and health care facilities**, The American Institute for Architects Press, Washington DC.
http://www.e-architect.com/pia/pubs/aah.asp

BANDOLIER 73, **Hospital-acquired infection**.
http://www.jr2.ox.ac.uk/bandolier/band73/b73-3.html

Barrie, D, Hoffman, PN, Wilson, JA and Kramer, JM (1994), *Contamination of hospital linen by* Bacillus cereus, **Journal of Epidemiology and Infection**, Vol 113, pp 297–306.

Barrie, D (1994), *How hospital linen and laundry services are provided*, **Journal of Hospital Infection**, Vol 27 No 3, July, pp 219–235.

Birch, BR, Perera, BS, Hyde, WA, Ruehorn, V, Ganguli, LA, Kramer, JM and Turnbull, PCB (1981), Bacillus cereus *cross-infection in a maternity unit*, **Journal of Hospital Infection**, Vol 2, pp 349–354.

Borau, J, Czap, R, Strellrecht, K and Venezia, R (2000), *Long-term control of Legionella species in potable water after a nosocomial legionnelosis outbreak in an intensive care unit*, **Infection Control and Hospital Epidemiology**, Vol 21 No 9, September, pp 602–603.
http://www.slackinc.com/general/iche/stor0900/09cc2.htm

Brundrett, GW (1992), **Legionella and Building Services**, Butterworth-Heinemann, Oxford.

Brunton, WA (1995), *Infection and hospital laundry*, **Lancet**, Vol 345 No 8964, 17 June, pp 1574–1575.

CDC (2001), Healthcare Infection Control Practices Advisory Committee (HICPAC), **Draft guidelines for environmental infection control in healthcare facilities**
http://www.cdc.gov/ncidod/hip/enviro/env_guide_draft.pdf.

Collinge, J (1999), *Variant Creutzfeldt–Jakob disease*, **Lancet**, Vol 354 No 9175, 24 July, pp 317–323.

Cowan, ME, Allen, J and Pilkington, F (1995), *Small dishwashers for hospital ward kitchens*, **Journal of Hospital Infection**, Vol 29 No 3, March, pp 227–231.

Dandalides, PC, Rutala, WA and Sarubbi, FA Jr (1984), *Postoperative infections following cardiac surgery: association with an environmental reservoir in a cardiothoracic intensive care unit*, **Infection Control**, Vol 5, pp 378–384.

Donaldson, LJ and Donaldson, RJ (2000), **Essential Public Health**, 2nd edition, LibraPharm Limited, Newbury.

Dryden, MS, Keyworth, N, Gabb, R and Stein, K (1994), *Asymptomatic food handlers as the source of nosocomial salmonellosis*, **Journal of Hospital Infection**, Vol 28 No 3, November, pp 195–208.

Dyson C, Ribeiro, CD and Westmoreland, D (1995), *Large scale use of ciprofloxacin in hospitals in the control of a Salmonella outbreak in a hospital for the mentally handicapped*. **Journal of Hospital Infection**, Vol 29 No 4, April, pp 287–296.

Fuell, WG (1987), *Developments in linen services: modern laundry design considerations*, **Hospital Engineer**, Vol 41 No 4, April, pp 3–6.

Gardner, J and Peel, M (1991), **Introduction to Sterilization, Disinfection and Infection**, 2nd edition, Churchill-Livingstone, Melbourne.

Goldthorpe, G, Kerry, P and Drabu, YJ (1991), *Refrigerated food storage in hospital ward areas*, **Journal of Hospital Infection**, Vol 18 No 1, May, pp 63–66.

Gupta, AK, Anand, NK, Manmohan, A, Lamba, IM, Gupta, R and Srivastava, L (1991), *Role of bacteriological monitoring of the hospital environment and medical equipment in a neo-natal intensive care unit*, **Journal of Hospital Infection**, Vol 19 No 4, December, pp 263–271.

Harbeth, S, Sudre, P, Dharan, S, Cadenas, M and Pittet, D (1999), *Outbreak of* Enterobacter cloacae *related to under-staffing, overcrowding and poor hygiene practices*, **Infection Control Hospital Epidemiology**, Vol 20 No 9, September, pp 598–603.

Hempshall, P and Thomson, M (1998), *Dirt alert*, **Nursing Times**, Vol 94, pp 63–64.

Horton, R (1995), *Hand washing: the fundamental infection control principle*, **British Journal of Nursing**, Vol 4 No 16, pp 926–933.

ICNA (1998), **Guidelines for Hand Hygiene**, ICNA/DEB Ltd, West Lothian.

Keyworth, N (2000), 'Introduction to microbiology and virology', in McCulloch, J (Ed), **Infection control: science management and practice**, Whurr Publishers, London, Chapter 2.

Larson, AP (1995), *Infection control guidelines for infection control practice, APIC Guidelines for handwashing and hand antisepsis in healthcare settings*, **American Journal of Infection Control**, Vol 23, pp 251–269.

Laurenson, IF, Whyte, AS, Fox, C and Babb, JR (1999), *Contaminated surgical instruments and variant Creutzfeldt-Jakob disease*, **Lancet**, Vol 354 No 9192, 20 November, p 1823.
http://www.thelancet.com/

Loudon, KW, Coke, AP, Burnie, JP, Shaw, AJ, Oppenheim, BA and Morris, CQ (1996), *Kitchens as a source of* Aspergillus niger *infection*, **Journal of Hospital Infection**, Vol 32 No 3, March, pp 191–198.

Maguire, H, Pharoah, P, Walsh, B, Davison, C, Barrie, D, Threlfall, EJ and Chambers, S (2000), *Hospital outbreak of* Salmonella virchow *possibly associated with a food handler*, **Journal of Hospital Infection**, Vol 44 No 4, April, pp 261–266.

Marshall, BE, Sen, RA, Chadwick, PR and Keaney, MGL (1997), 'Environmental contamination of a new general surgical ward', Presentation at the Federation of Infection Societies in Manchester, November.

Mayhall, GC (Ed) (1999), **Hospital Epidemiology and Infection Control**, 2nd Edition. Lippincott, Williams & Wilkins, Philadelphia, PA, ISBN 0683-306-081.

McManus, AT, Mason, AD Jr, McManus, WF and Pruitt, BA Jr (1994), *A decade of reduced gram negative infections and mortality associated with improved isolation of burned patients*, **Archives of Surgery**, Vol 129, pp 1306–1309.

Murphy, O, Gray, J, Gordon, S and Bint, AJ (1995), *An outbreak of campylobacter food poisoning in a health care setting*, **Journal of Hospital Infection**, Vol 30 No 3, July, pp 225–228.

Redpath, C and Farrington, M (1997), *Dispose of disposables?*, **Journal of Hospital Infection**, Vol 35 No 4, April, pp 313–317.

Regan, CM, Syed, O and Turnstall, PJ (1995), *A hospital outbreak of* Clostridium perfringens *food poisoning – implications for food hygiene review in hospitals*, **Journal of Hospital Infection**, Vol 29 No 1, January, pp 69–73.

Richards, J, Parr, E and Riseborough, P (1993), *Hospital food hygiene: the application of Hazard Analysis Critical Control points to conventional hospital catering*, **Journal of Hospital Infection**, Vol 24 No 4, August, pp 273–282.

Viral Gastro Enteritis Sub Committee of the PHLS Virology Committee, *Outbreaks of gastro enteritis associated with SRSVs*, **PHLS Microbiology Digest**, Vol 10 No 1.

Wall, PG, Ryan, MJ, Warp, LR and Rowe, B (1996), *Outbreak of salmonellosis in hospitals in England and Wales 1992–1994*, **Journal of Hospital Infection**, Vol 33 No 3, July; pp 181–190.

Weernink, A, Severin, WP, Tjernberg, I and Drskshoorn, L (1995), *Pillows, an unexpected source of Acinetobacter*, **Journal of Hospital Infection**, Vol 29 No 3, March, pp 189–199.

Wilcox, MH and Jones, BL (1995), *Enterococci and hospital laundry*, **Lancet**, 4 March, Vol 345 No 8949, p 594.

Zilz, MA (1982), *Relation of the inanimate hospital environment to endemic nosocomial infection*, **The New England Journal of Medicine**, Vol 307 No 25, 16 December, pp 1562–1566.

Infection control in specialist settings – literature review

FACILITIES FOR CRITICAL CARE

- Intensive care unit

- High dependency unit

- Coronary care unit

- Paediatric intensive care unit

- Special care baby unit

NHS Estates publications

HBN 57: Critical care facilities, The Stationery Office, 2002.

HTM 2025: Ventilation in healthcare premises, HMSO, 1994.

Department of Health publications

Expert Group (1999), **Comprehensive critical care: a review of adult critical care services**.
http://www.doh.gov.uk/pdfs/criticalcare.pdf

NHS Executive (2000), HSC 2000/017: 'Modernising critical care services'.
http://tap.ccta.gov.uk/doh/coin4.nsf/d06aa2d76da4c1d
6002568560064952b/3932656d15f1e34a002568e9003
3ad5e/$FILE/017hsc.pdf

NHS Executive South East Regional Office press release (2000), 'NHS winter plans go into top gear as Minister unveils a major boost to critical care bed numbers and an additional £62m for step down care'.
http://www.doh.gov.uk/stheast/press110.htm

Other publications

Archibald, LK, Manning, ML, Bell, LM, Banerjee, S and Jarvis, WR (1997), *Patient density, nurse-to-patient ratio and nosocomial infection risk in a pediatric cardiac intensive care unit*, **Pediatric Infectious Disease Journal**, Vol 16 No 11, November, pp 1045–1050.
http://www.lww.com/PIDJ/0891-366811-97toc.html

Audit Commission (1999) **Critical to success: the place of efficient and effective critical care services within the acute hospital**, Audit Commission Publications, Wetherby.
http://www.audit-commission.gov.uk/ac2/NR/Health/
brccare.htm

Bonten, MJ, Hayden, MK, Nathan, C, van Voorhis, J, Matushek, M, Slaughter, S, Rice, T and Weinstein, RA (1996), *Epidemiology of colonisation of patients and environment with vancomycin-resistant enterococci*, **Lancet**, Vol 348 No 9042, 14 December, pp 1615–1619.

Eckmanns, T, Rath, A, Rüden, H, Gastmeier, P and Daschner, F (2000), *Outbreak of* Enterobacter cloacae *related to understaffing, overcrowding, and poor hygiene practices*, **Infection Control and Hospital Epidemiology**, Vol 21, pp 305–306.

Gupta, AK, Anand, NK, Manmohan, IMS, Lamba, R, Gupta, L and Srivastava, L (1991), *Role of bacteriological monitoring of the hospital environment and medical equipment in a neonatal intensive care unit*, **Journal of Hospital Infection**, Vol 19 No 4, pp 263–271.

Harvey, MA (1998), *Critical care unit bedside design and furnishings: impact on nosocomial infections*, **Infection Control and Hospital Epidemiology**, Vol 19 No 8, pp 597–601.

Haley, RW and Bregman, DA (1982), *The role of under staffing, over crowding in recurrent outbreaks of Staphylococcal infection in a neo-natal special care unit*, **Journal of Infectious Diseases**, Vol 145 No 6, June, pp 875–885.

Health Service Journal (2000), *Intermediate care model more expensive*, Vol 110, pp 5722–5725.

Health Technology Assessment (2000), *Outcome measures for adult critical care: a systematic review*, Vol 4 No 24.
http://www.hta.nhsweb.nhs.uk/fullmono/mon424.pdf

Intensive Care Society (ICS) (2000), *Comments on HBN 27: Intensive Therapy Unit: The formal response to NHS Estates 03/02/00.*

Leroyer, A, Bedu, A, Lombrail, P, Desplanques, L, Diakite, B, Bingen, E, Aujard, Y and Brodin, M (1997), *Prolongation of hospital stay and extra costs due to hospital acquired infection in a neo-natal unit*, **Journal of Hospital Infection**, Vol 35 No 1, January, pp 37–45.
http://www.harcourt-international.com/journals/jhin/
previous.cfm?art=hi960127

Lyons, R, Wareham, K, Hutchings, H, Major, E and Ferguson, B (2000), *Population requirements for adult critical care beds: a prospective quantitative and qualitative study*, **Lancet**, Vol 355, pp 595–598.

McGucken, MB and Kelsen, SG (1981), *Surveillance in a surgical intensive care unit: patient and environment*, **Infection Control**, Vol 2 No 1, January–February, pp 21–25.

National Audit Office (2000), **Report by the Comptroller and Auditor General: The Management and Control of Hospital-acquired Infection in Acute NHS Trusts in England**, The Stationery Office, London.

O'Connell, NH and Humphreys, H (2000), *Intensive care unit design and environmental factors in the acquisition of infection*, **Journal of Hospital Infection**, Vol 45 No 4, August, pp 255–262.
http://www.harcourt-international.com/journals/jhin/previous.cfm?art=jhin.2000.0768

Oelberg, D, Joyner, S, Jiang, X, Laborde, D, Islam, MP and Pickering, LK (2000), *Detection of pathogen transmission in neonatal nurseries using DNA markers as surrogate indicators*, **Pediatrics**, Vol 105 No 2, February, pp 311–315.
http://www.pediatrics.org/cgi/content/abstract/105/2/311

Risi, GF and Tomascak, V (1998), *Prevention of infection in the immunocompromised host*, **American Journal of Infection Control**, Vol 26 No 6, pp 594–606.

Robert, R, Fridkin, SK, Blumberg, HM, Anderson, B, White, N, Ray, SM, Chan, J and Jarvis, WR (2000), *The influence of the composition of the nursing staff on primary bloodstream infection rates in a surgical intensive care unit*, **Infection Control and Hospital Epidemiology**, Vol 21 No 1, January.
http://www.slackinc.com/general/iche/stor0100/1rob.htm

Shahani, AK (2000), **How many beds in a critical care unit?** Institute of Modelling for Healthcare and Practical Insights Ltd, Southampton.
http://www.doh.gov.uk/compcritcare/critcare/

Steiner, A, Vaughan, B and Hanford, L (1999), **Intermediate care: shifting the money**, Kings Fund, London.
http://www.kingsfund.org.uk/eHealthSocialCare/html/rehab_publications.html

CLINICAL WARD AREAS

- Surgical ward

- Medical ward

- Emergency admission unit

- Elderly care unit

- Paediatric ward

- Isolation facilities

Including:

- Catering facilities

- Laundry facilities

- Waste disposal facilities

Acts and Regulations

Carriage of Dangerous Goods by Road Regulations 1996, SI 2095, HMSO.
http://www.hmso.gov.uk/si/si1996/Uksi_19962095_en_1.htm

Control of Pollution (Amendment) Act 1989. HMSO
http://www.hmso.gov.uk/acts/acts1989/Ukpga_19890014_en_1.htm

The Controlled Waste (Amendment) Regulations 1993, SI 566, HMSO.
http://www.hmso.gov.uk/si/si1993/Uksi_19930566_en_1.htm

Environment Act 1995. HMSO.
http://www.hmso.gov.uk/acts/acts1995/Ukpga_19950025_en_1.htm

Environmental Protection Act 1990. The Stationery Office.
http://www.hmso.gov.uk/acts/acts1990/Ukpga_19900043_en_1.htm

The Environmental Protection (Duty of Care) Regulations, SI 1991 No 2839, HMSO.
http://www.hmso.gov.uk/si/si1991/Uksi_19912839_en_1.htm

Food Safety (General Food Hygiene) Regulations 1995, SI 1763, HMSO.
http://www.hmso.gov.uk/si/si1995/Uksi_19951763_en_1.htm

Food Safety (Temperature Control) Regulations 1995, SI 2200, HMSO.
http://www.hmso.gov.uk/si/si1995/Uksi_19952200_en_1.htm

The Special Waste (Amendment) Regulations 1997, SI 251, HMSO.
http://www.hmso.gov.uk/si/si1997/97025101.htm

NHS Estates publications

HBN 02: The whole hospital: briefing and operational policy, HMSO, 1993.

HBN 04: In-patient accommodation: options for choice, HMSO, 1997.

HBN 10: Catering department, HMSO, 1997.

HBN 23: Hospital accommodation for children and young people, HMSO, 1994.

HBN 25: Laundry, HMSO, 1994.

HBN 40: Common activity spaces (Vol 1 Public areas, Vol 2 Treatment areas, Vol 3 Staff areas, Vol 4 Circulation areas), 1995.

HTM 2023: Access and accommodation for engineering services, HMSO, 1995.

HTM 2022: Medical gas pipeline systems, HMSO, 1997.

HTM 2025: Ventilation in healthcare premises: design considerations, HMSO, 1994.

HTM 2027: Hot and cold water supply, storage and mains service, HMSO, 1995.

HTM 2040: The control of Legionella in healthcare premises – a code of practice, HMSO, 1994.

HTM 2075: Clinical waste disposal/treatment technologies (alternatives to incineration), HMSO, 1998.

HGN. "Safe" hot water and surface temperatures, HMSO, 1998.

HGN. Safe disposal of clinical waste: whole hospital policy, HMSO, 1995.

HGN. Clinical waste incineration joint venture arrangements, HMSO, 1994.

Better by design, 1994.
http://www.nhsestates.gov.uk/download/better_by_design.pdf

Design guide – the design of community hospitals, HMSO, 1991.

Environments for quality care, HMSO, 1994.

A strategic guide to clinical waste management for general managers and chief executives, HMSO, 1994.

Department of Health publications

Food handlers: fitness to work – guidelines for food business managers, HMSO, 1996.

A guide to food hazards and your business, 1996.
http://www.doh.gov.uk/busguide/foodsafe/fdhbch.htm

A guide to the General Food Hygiene Regulations 1995.
http://www.doh.gov.uk/busguide/hygrc.htm

Hospital catering: delivering a quality service, NHS Executive, HMSO, 1996.

Hospital laundry arrangements for used and infected linen, HSG(95)18, 1995.

Management of outbreaks of food-borne illness, HMSO, 1994.

Pest control management for the health service, HMSO, 1992.

Other publications

Audit Commission (1997), **Getting sorted: the safe and economic management of hospital waste**, Audit Commission Publications, ISBN 1-86240-017-2.
http://www.audit-commission.gov.uk/ac2/NR/Health/ebnh0397.htm

Barrie, D (1994), *How hospital linen and laundry services are provided*, **Journal of Hospital Infection**, Vol 27 No 3, July, pp 219–235.

Barrie, D (1998), *Central Sterilising Club – Laundry Working Group, Discussion Paper*, **CSC Bulletin**, Vol 3 No 1.

Birch, BR and Perera, BS et al (1981), Bacillus cereus *cross-infection in a maternity unit*, **Journal of Hospital Infection**, Vol 2, pp 349–354.

Brunton, G (1995), *Infection and hospital laundry*, **Lancet**, Vol 345 No 8964, 17 June, pp 1574–1575.

Cartmill, TDI, Panigrahi, H, Worsley, MA, McCann, DC, Nice, CN and Keith, E (1994), *Management and control of a large outbreak of diarrhoea due to* Clostridium difficile, **Journal of Hospital Infection**, Vol 27, pp 1–15.

Food Safety (General Food Hygiene) Regulations 1995: Industry guide to good hygiene practice: catering guide, ISBN 0 900 103 00 0, Chadwick House Group Ltd Publications Department, Chadwick Court, 15 Hatfields, London SE1 8DJ.

Health and Safety Executive (1994), **Workroom temperatures in places where food is handled** (Food sheet no 3).
http://www.hse.gov.uk/pubns/food3.htm

Health Services Advisory Committee and the Environment Agency (1999), **Safe disposal of clinical waste**, ISBN 0-7176-2492-7, HSE Books.

Keys, A, Baldwin, A and Austin, S (2000), *Reducing waste by design*, **Building Services Journal**, December, pp 49–50.

Martin, M (1991), **The need for single rooms in the care of general acute patients**, Medical Architecture Research Unit, Polytechnic of North London.

Otero, RB (1997), **Healthcare textile services: infection control**, Professional Development Series, Chicago, IL, January, pp 1–13.

Ramm, AE et al (1996), *An outbreak of fatal nosocomial infections due to group A Streptococcus on a medical ward*, **Infection Control and Hospital Epidemiology**, Vol 7, 17 July, pp 429–431.

Wall, PG, Ryan, MJ, Warp, LR and Rowe, B (1996), *Outbreak of salmonellosis in hospitals in England and Wales 1992–1994*, **Journal of Hospital Infection**, Vol 33 No 3, July, pp 181–190.

Wilcox, MH and Jones, BL (1995), *Enterococci and hospital laundry*, **Lancet**, 4 March, Vol 345 No 8949, p 594.

RENAL UNIT

NHS Estates publications

HBN 53: Satellite dialysis unit, HMSO, 1996.

Other publications

Arvantidou, M, Spaia, S, Velegraki, A, Pazarloglou, Id, Kanetidis, D, Pangidis, P, Askepidis, N, Katsinas, Ch, Vayonas, G and Katsouyannopoulos, V (2000), *High level of recovery of fungi from water and dialysate in haemodialysis units*, **Journal of Hospital Infection**, Vol 45 No 3, July, pp 225– 30. http://www.harcourt-international.com/journals/jhin/previous.cfm?art=jhin.2000.0763

Bergogne-Berezin, E (1995), *The increasing significance of outbreaks of Acinetobacter spp.: the need for control and new agents*, **Journal of Hospital Infection**, Vol 30 (Supplement), pp 441–452.

Ling, Jm, Wise, R, Woo, Th and Cheng, Af (1996), *Investigation of the epidemiology of hospital isolates of Acinetobacter anitratus by two molecular methods*, **Journal of Hospital Infection**, Vol 32 No 1, January, pp 29–38.

Morin, P (2000), *Identification of the bacteriological contamination of a water treatment line used for haemodialysis and its disinfection*, **Journal of Hospital Infection**, Vol 45 No 3, July, pp 218–224.

http://www.harcourt-international.com/journals/jhin/previous.cfm?art=jhin.2000.0732

The Renal Association (1997), **Treatment of adult patients with renal failure: recommended standards and audit measures**, November 2nd edition (prepared by the Standards Subcommittee of the Renal Association on behalf of the Renal Association and the Royal College of Physicians of London in collaboration with the British Transplantation Society and the Intensive Care Society).

Sessa, A, Meroni, M, Battini, G, Pitingolo, F, Gioradno, F, Marks, M and Casella, P (1996), *Nosocomial outbreak of Aspergillus fumigatus infection among patients in a renal unit*, **Nephrology Dialysis Transplantation**, Vol 11 No 7, July, pp 1322–1324. http://ndt.oupjournals.org/cgi/content/abstract/11/7/1322?

Stragier, A (1996), *Water treatment for haemodialysis: not as safe as anticipated*, **EDTNA/ERCA**, Vol 22 No 4, pp 12–14.

MATERNITY UNIT AND NEONATAL UNIT

NHS Estates publications

HBN 21: Maternity department, HMSO, 1996.

HBN 26: Operating department, HMSO, 1991.

Department of Health publications

Changing childbirth, part 1: report of the Expert Maternity Group, HMSO, 1993 ('Cumberlege report').

Other publications

British Paediatric Association (1994), **Guidelines for the establishment and operation of human milk banks in the UK** (now the Royal College of Paediatrics and Child Health).

Claesson, BE and Claesson, UL (1995), *An outbreak of endometritis in a maternity unit caused by spread of Group streptococci from a shower head*, **Journal of Hospital Infection**, Vol 6 No 3, pp 304–311.

Clinical Standards Advisory Group (1993), **Neonatal intensive care: access to and availability of specialist services**, HMSO.

Cotton, MF, Wasserman, E, Pieper, CH, Theron, DC, Van Tubbergh, D, Campbell, G, Fang, FC and Barnes, AJ (2000), *Invasive disease due to extended spectrum beta-lactamase-producing Klebsiella pneumoniae in a neonatal unit: the possible role of cockroaches*, **Journal of Hospital Infection**, Vol 44 No 1, January, pp 13–17. http://www.harcourt-international.com/journals/jhin/previous.cfm?art=jhin.1999.0650

Fujita, K and Murono, K (1996), *Nosocomial acquisition of* Escherichia coli *by infants delivered in hospitals*, **Journal of Hospital Infection**, Vol 32 No 4, April, pp 277–281.
http://www.harcourt-international.com/journals/jhin/previous.cfm?art=hi960033

Galloway, A, Noel, I, Efstratiou, A, Saint, E and White, DR (1994), *An outbreak of Group C streptococcal infection in a maternity unit*, **Journal of Hospital Infection**, Vol 28 No 1, September, pp 31–37.

Haynes, J, Anderson, AW and Spence, WN (1987), *An outbreak of puerperal fever caused by Group G streptococci*, **Journal of Hospital Infection**, Vol 9 No 2, March, pp 120–125.

National Association of Health Authorities and Trusts (NAHAT) (1995), **Safe and sound: security in NHS Maternity Units**.

Oelberg, D, Joyner, S, Jiang, X, Laborde, D, Islam, MP and Pickering, LK (2000), *Detection of pathogen transmission in neonatal nurseries using DNA markers as surrogate indicators*, **Pediatrics**, Vol 105 No 2, February, pp 311–315.
http://www.pediatrics.org/cgi/content/abstract/105/2/311

Teare, EL, Smithson, RD, Efstratiou, A, Devenish, WR and Noah, ND (1989), *An outbreak of puerperal fever caused by Group C streptococci*, **Journal of Hospital Infection**, Vol 13 No 4, May, pp 337–347.

ONCOLOGY UNIT/BURNS UNIT

NHS Estates publications

HTM 2025:Ventilation in healthcare premises:

Design considerations, HMSO, 1994.

Operational management, HMSO, 1994.

Validation and verification, HMSO, 1994.

HTM 2040: The control of Legionella in healthcare premises: a code of practice:

Design considerations, HMSO, 1994.

Good practice guide, HMSO, 1994.

Management policy, HMSO, 1994.

Operational management, HMSO, 1994.

Validation and verification, HMSO, 1994.

Other publications

Bretagne, S, Bart-Delabesse, E, Wechsler, J, Kuentz, M, Dhédin, N and Cordonnier, C (1997), *Fatal primary cutaneous aspergillosis in a bone marrow transplant recipient: nosocomial acquisition in a laminar-air flow room*, **Journal of Hospital Infection**, Vol 36 No 3, July, pp 235–239.
http://www.harcourt-international.com/journals/jhin/previous.cfm?art=hi970229

Chloe, LT, Smith, D, Merz, WG, Streifel, AJ, Bova, G, Gay, L, Miller, CB and Perl, TM (2000), *Refinements of environmental assessment during an outbreak investigation of invasive aspergillosis in a leukemia and bone marrow transplant unit*, **Infection Control and Hospital Epidemiology**, Vol 21 No 1, January, pp 18–23.
http://www.slackinc.com/general/iche/stor0100/1thi.htm

Cornet, M, Levy, V, Fleury, L, Lortholary, J, Barquins, S, Coureul, MH, Deliere, E, Zittoun, R, Brücker, G and Bouvet, A (1999), *Efficacy of prevention by high efficiency particulate air filtration or laminar airflow against aspergillus airborne contamination during hospital renovation*, **Infection Control and Hospital Epidemiology**, Vol 20 No 7, July, pp 508–513.
http://www.slackinc.com/general/iche/stor0799/cor.htm

Denton, M, Hawkey, PM, Hoy, CM and Porter, C (1993), *Co-existent cross infection with* streptococcus pneumoniae *and Group B streptococci on an adult oncology unit*, **Journal of Hospital Infection**, Vol 23 No 4, April, pp 271–278.

Gardner, C (1994), *An outbreak of hospital-acquired cryptosporidiosis*, **British Journal of Nursing**, Vol 3 No 4, 24 February–9 March, pp 152–154.

Gerba, CP, Rose, JB and Haas, CN (1996), *Sensitive populations: who is at the greatest risk?*, **International Journal of Food Microbiology**, Vol 30, pp 113–123.

Gruteke, P, Van Belkum, A, Schouls, LM, Hendriks, WDH, Reubsaet, FA, Dokter, J, Boxma, H and Verbrugh, HA (1996), *Outbreak of Group A streptococci in a burn centre: use of pheno- and genotypic procedures for strain tracking*, **Journal of Clinical Microbiology**, Vol 34 No 1, January, pp 114–118.
http://jcm.asm.org/cgi/reprint/34/1/114.pdf

Hedin, G and Hambraeus, A (1991), *Multiply antibiotic-resistant* Staphylococcus epidermidis *in patients, staff and environment – a one week survey in a bone marrow transplant unit*, **Journal of Hospital Infection**, Vol 17, pp 95–106.

Mahieu, LM, De dooy, JJ, Van Laer, FA, Jansens, H and Ieven, MM (2000), *A prospective study on factors influencing aspergillus spore load in the air during renovation works in a neonatal intensive care unit*, **Journal of Hospital Infection**, Vol 45 No 3, July, pp 191–197.

http://www.harcourt-international.com/journals/jhin/previous.cfm?art=jhin.2000.0773

Manuel, R and Kibbler, C (1998), *The epidemiology and prevention of invasive aspergillosis*, **Journal of Hospital Infection**, Vol 39 No 2, June, pp 95–109. http://www.harcourt-international.com/journals/jhin/previous.cfm?art=hi980365

Morris, G, Kokki, MH, Anderson, K and Richardson, MD (2000), *Sampling of aspergillus spores in air*, **Journal of Hospital Infection**, Vol 44 No 2, February, pp 81–92. http://www.harcourt-international.com/journals/jhin/previous.cfm?art=jhin.1999.0688

Murphy, OM and Gould, FK (1999), *Prevention of nosocomial infection in solid organ transplantation*, **Journal of Hospital Infection**, Vol 42 No 3, July, pp 177–183 (review). http://www.harcourt-international.com/journals/jhin/previous.cfm?art=jhin.1999.0599

O'Dea, TJ (1996), *Protecting the immunocompromised patient: the role of the hospital clinical engineer*, **Journal Clinical Engineer**, Vol 21 No 6, Nov–Dec, pp 466–482.

Ravn, P, Lundgren, JD, Kjaeldgaard, P, Holten-Anderson, W, Hjlyng, N, Nielsen, Jo and Gaub, J (1992), *Nosocomial outbreak of eryplosporidiosis in AIDS patients*, **British Medical Journal**, 302, January, pp 277–280.

Ridgeway, EJ and Allen, KD (1993), *Clustering of Group A streptococcal infection on a burns unit: important lessons in outbreak management*, **Journal of Hospital Infection**, Vol 25 No 3, November, pp 173–182.

Risi, GF and Tomascak, V (1998), *Prevention of infection in the immunocompromised host*, **American Journal of Infection Control**, Vol 26 No 6, pp 594–606.

Rogers, TR and Barnes, RA (1988), *Prevention of airborne fungal infection in immunocompromised patients*, **Journal of Hospital Infection**, Vol 11 (supplement A), pp 15–20.

Williams, PL (2000), *Fungus among us – fighting fungal infection during construction*, **Health Facilities Management**, March, pp 39–44.

Withington, S, Chambers, ST, Beard, ME, Inder, A, Allen, JR, Ikram, RB, Schousboe, MI, Heaton, DC, Spearing, RI, Hart, DNJ (1998), *Invasive aspergillosis in severely neutropenic patients over 18 years: impact of intranasal amphotericin B and HEPA filtration*, **Journal of Hospital Infection**, Vol 38, pp 11–18. http://www.harcourt-international.com/journals/jhin/previous.cfm?art=hi970317

FACILITIES FOR SURGICAL PROCEDURES

- Day Surgery Unit

- Operating Theatres

- Surgery in General Practice and minor operations or invasive treatments by professions allied to medicine (Chiropody, Acupuncture, Dental Surgery etc)

- Endoscopy

- Medical investigation and treatment centres

NHS Estates publications

HBN 13: Sterile services department, HMSO, 1993.

HBN 21: Maternity department, HMSO, 1996.

HBN 22: Accident and emergency facilities for adults and children, The Stationery Office, 2002.

HBN 26: Operating department, HMSO, 1991.

HBN 36: Vol 1: Local healthcare facilities, HMSO, 1995.

Vol 2: Local healthcare facilities – case studies, HMSO, 1996.

Sup 1: Accommodation for professions allied to medicine, HMSO, 1997.

HBN 52: Vol 1: Accommodation for day care: Day Surgery Unit, HMSO, 1993.

Sup 1. Day Surgery: review of schedules of accommodation, HMSO, 1997.

Vol 2: Accommodation for day care: Endoscopy Unit, HMSO, 1994.

Vol 3: Accommodation for day care: Medical Investigation and Treatment Unit, HMSO, 1995.

HTM 2022: Medical gas pipeline systems, HMSO, 1997.

HTM 2025: Ventilation in healthcare premises:

Management policy, HMSO, 1994.

Design considerations, HMSO, 1994.

Validation and verification, HMSO, 1994.

Operational management, HMSO, 1994.

HFN 8: Minimal access therapy, HMSO, 1996.

Other publications

Holton, J and Ridgway, GL (1993), *Commissioning operating theatres*, **Journal of Hospital Infection**, Vol 23, pp 161–167.

Holton, J, Ridgway, GL and Reynoldstone, AJ (1990), *A microbiologist's view of commissioning operating theatres*, **Journal of Hospital Infection**, Vol 16 No 1, July, pp 29–34.

Humphreys, H (1993), *Infection control and the design of a new operating suite*, **Journal of Hospital Infection**, Vol 23 No 1, pp 61–70.

Sanchez, RO and Hernandez, JM (1999), *Infection control during construction and renovation in the operating room*, **Semin Perioperative Nursing**, October, Vol 8 No 4, pp 208–214.

DIAGNOSTIC IMAGING FACILITIES

NHS Estates publications

HBN 6: Facilities for diagnostic imaging and interventional radiology, The Stationery Office, 2002.

PATHOLOGY, MORTUARY AND POST-MORTEM ROOMS

NHS Estates publications

HBN 15: Accommodation for pathology services, HMSO, 1991.

HBN 20: Facilities for mortuary and post-mortem room services, The Stationery Office, 2001.

Acts and Regulations

Control of Substances Hazardous to Health (COSHH) Regulations (1999), SI 1999 No. 437, The Stationery Office.
http://www.hmso.gov.uk/si/si1999/19990437.htm

Other publications

Brassil, KE and Zilman, MA (1993), *Design for a hospital mortuary*, **Pathology**, October; Vol 25 No 4, pp 333–337.

Health Service Advisory Committee (1991), **Safe working and the prevention of infection in clinical laboratories**, HMSO, ISBN 0-11-885446-1.

Health Service Advisory Committee (1991), **Safety in Health Services Laboratories: Safe working and the prevention of infection in the mortuary and post mortem room**, ISBN 0-11-885448-8.

Ironside, JW and Bell, JE (1996), *The 'high risk' neuropathological autopsy in AIDS and Creutzfeldt–Jakob disease: principles and practice*, **Neuropathol Appl Neurobiol**, October, Vol 22 No 5, pp 388–393.

ACCIDENT AND EMERGENCY UNIT

NHS Estates publications

HBN 22: Accident and emergency facilities for adults and children, The Stationery Office, 2002.

OUT-PATIENT FACILITIES

NHS Estates publications

HBN 12: Out-patients department:

>   Supplement 1 – Genito-Urinary Medicine Clinics, HMSO, 1990.

>   Supplement 2 – Oral Surgery, Orthodontics, Restorative Dentistry, HMSO, 1993.

>   Supplement 3 – ENT and Audiology Clinics, Hearing Aid Centre, HMSO, 1993.

>   Supplement 4 – Ophthalmology, HMSO, 1996.

HFN 14: Disability access, HMSO, 1996.

HBN 22: Accident and emergency facilities for adults and children, The Stationery Office, 2002.

Other publications

Herwaldt, LA, Smith, SD and Carter, CD (1998), *Infection control in the out-patient setting*, **Infection Control and Hospital Epidemiology**, January, Vol 19 No 1, pp 41–74.

Goodman, RA and Solomon, SI (1991), *Transmission of infectious disease in out-patient healthcare settings*, **JAMA**, Vol 265, pp 2377–2381.

NHS Accident and Emergency Departments in England: report by the Comptroller and Auditor General, National Audit Office, HMSO, 1992.

NHS Walk-in Centres – an introduction, 21733 2P May 2000 (BAB).

PROFESSIONS ALLIED TO MEDICINE

- Physiotherapy

- Occupational Therapy

- Hydrotherapy

- Speech Therapy

NHS Estates publications

HBN 8: Facilities for rehabilitation services, The Stationery Office, 2000.

HBN 12 Supplement 3 – ENT and audiology clinics, hearing aid centre, HMSO, 1993.

HBN 36: Local healthcare facilities. Supplement 1 – accommodation for professions allied to medicine, HMSO, 1997.

Other publications

Aspinall, ST and Graham, R (1989), *Two sources of contamination of a hydrotherapy pool by environmental organisms*, **Journal of Hospital Infection**, Vol 14, pp 285–292.

Public Health Laboratory Service, **Hygiene for hydrotherapy pools**, 2nd ed, PHLS, London, 1999 (ISBN 090-1144-460).

STERILE SERVICES DEPARTMENTS

NHS Estates publications

HBN 13: Sterile services department, HMSO, 1993.

HTM 2010: Sterilization:

Part 1 Management policy, HMSO, 1994.

Part 2 Design considerations, HMSO, 1995.

Part 3 Validation and verification, HMSO, 1995.

Part 4 and 6 Operational management (new edition) with testing and validation protocols, HMSO, 1997.

Part 5 Good practice guide, HMSO, 1995.

HTM 2030: Washer-disinfectors:

Operational management, HMSO, 1997

Design considerations, HMSO, 1997.

Validation and verificatiON, HMSO, 1997.

HTM 2031 Clean steam for sterilization, HMSO, 1997.

Department of Health publications

'Decontamination of medical devices', HSC 2000/032 http://www.doh.gov.uk/coinh.htm

Other publications

Institute of Sterile Services Management, **Quality standards and recommended practices for Sterile Services Departments**, ISSM, 1998.

DECONTAMINATION GUIDANCE

NHS Estates publications

HBN 13: Sterile services department, HMSO, 1993.

HTM 2010: Sterilization:

Part 1 Management policy, HMSO, 1994.

Part 2 Design considerations, HMSO, 1995.

Part 3 Validation and verification, HMSO, 1995.

Part 4 and 6 Operational management (new edition) with testing and validation protocols, HMSO, 1997.

Part 5 Good practice guide, HMSO, 1995.

HTM 2025: Ventilation in healthcare premises:

Management policy, HMSO, 1994.

Design considerations, HMSO, 1994.

Validation and verification, HMSO, 1994.

Operational management, HMSO, 1994.

HTM 2030: Washer-disinfectors:

Operational management, HMSO, 1997

Design considerations, HMSO, 1997.

Validation and verification, HMSO, 1997.

HTM 2031: Clean steam for sterilization, HMSO, 1997.

Department of Health publications

Advisory Committee on Dangerous Pathogens/Spongiform Encephalopathy Advisory Committee (1998), **Transmissible Spongiform Encephalopathy Agents: Safe Working and the Prevention of Infection**.

Decontamination Programme Technical Manual – Part 1: Process Assessment Tool and Decontamination Guidance (updated), 2001. http://www.nhsestates.gov.uk/facilities_management/index.asp?submenu_ID=decontamination

Decontamination Programme Technical Manual – Part 2: Decontamination Organisational Review Information System (DORIS). http://www.nhsestates.gov.uk/facilities_management/index.asp?submenu_ID=decontamination

HSG(93)26 – 'Decontamination of Equipment prior to Inspection, Service or Repair'.

Medical Devices Agency publications

Device Bulletin DB9607 **Decontamination of Endoscopes.**

Device Bulletin DB9605 **The Purchase, Operation and Maintenance of Benchtop Steam Sterilisers.**

Device Bulletin DV9804 **The Validation and Periodic Testing of Benchtop Vacuum Steam Sterilisers.**

Safety Notice SN9619 – 'Compatibility of medical devices and their accessories and reprocessing units with cleaning, disinfecting and sterilising agents'.

Safety Notice SN 2002 (01) – 'Reporting adverse incidents and disseminating safety warnings'.

Single use medical devices: Implications and consequences of reuse.

Sterilisation, disinfection and cleaning of medical equipment: Parts 1,2 and 3.

Other publications

Ayliffe, GA (2000), *Decontamination of minimally invasive surgical endoscopes and accessories*, **Journal of Hospital Infection**, Vol 45 pp 263–277. http://www.harcourt-international.com/journals/jhin/previous.cfm?art=jhin.2000.0767

Institute of Sterile Services Management (1998), **Quality standards and recommended practices for sterile services departments**.

Smyth, ET, Mcilvenny, G, Thompson, IM, Adams, RJ, Mcbride, L, Young, B, Mitchell, E and Macauley, D (1999), *Sterilisation and disinfection in general practice in Northern Ireland*, **Journal of Hospital Infection**, October, Vol 43 No 23, pp 155–161.

Turala, WA and Weber, DJ (1999), *Infection control: the role of disinfection and sterilisation*, **Journal of Hospital Infection**, Vol 43 (Supplement), pp 343–355.

PHARMACY

NHS Estates publications

HBN 29: Accommodation for pharmaceutical services, HMSO, 1997.

SUPPLIES

NHS Estates publications

HFN 29: Materials management (supply, storage and distribution) in healthcare facilities, HMSO, 1998.

COMMUNITY AND PRIMARY CARE TRUSTS

- Nursing and residential homes

- Intermediate care facilities

- Hospice

- Primary care trust inpatient beds

Acts and Regulations

Statutory Instrument 1996 No. 2987, **The Disability Discrimination Code of Practice (Goods, Services,** **Facilities and Premises) Order 1996**, The Staionery Office. http://www.hmso.gov.uk/si/si1996/Uksi_19962987_en_1.htm

NHS Estates publications

HFN 19: The design of residential care and nursing homes for older people, NHS Estates/Centre for Accessible Environments, HMSO, 1998.

Design guide – The design of community hospitals, HMSO, 1991.

Department of Health publications

Private hospitals, homes and clinics registered under Section 23 of the Registered Homes Act 1984, ISBN 1-858-39868-1.

Other publications

Centre for Policy on Aging (1996), **A better home life: a code of practice for residential and nursing home care.**

Residential Forum National Institute for Social Work (1996), **Creating a home from home: a guide to standards.**

Royal College of General Practitioners Occasional Paper 43 (1990), **Community hospitals: preparing for the future.**

Public Health Medicine Environmental Group (PHMEG) (1995), **Guidelines on the Control of Infection in Residential and Nursing Homes**, London.

Worsley, MA, Ward, KA, Privett, S, Parker, L and Roberts, JM (1994), **Infection Control: a community perspective**, Cambridge Infection Control Nurses Association.

PRIMARY CARE PRACTICES

NHS Estates publications

HBN 12: Out-patients departments – Supplement 2: oral surgery, orthodontics, restorative surgery, HMSO, 1993.

HBN 36: Local healthcare facilities, HMSO, 1995.

General Medical Practice Premises – A Commentary – a guide to size, design and construction of GP premises (2002). http://www.nhsestates.gov.uk/capital_procurement/content/primary_care.html

General Medical Practice Premises – A Commentary – a guide to the provision of leasehold premises for GP occupation (2002). http://www.nhsestates.gov.uk/capital_procurement/content/primary_care.html

Department of Health publications

North West Regional Health Authority (1996), **Designing primary healthcare premises: a resource**
http://tap.ccta.gov.uk/doh/point.nsf/page/
3B0F33DAB001CAA30025661800674BC1?Open
Document

NURSERY AND CRECHE

Acts and Regulations

Children Act 1989, HMSO.
http://www.hmso.gov.uk/acts/acts1989/Ukpga_
19890041_en_1.htm

NHS Estates publications

HBN 23: Hospital accommodation for children and young people, HMSO, 1994.

Design Guide: The design of day nurseries with particular reference to district general hospitals, HMSO, 1991.

ACCOMMODATION FOR PEOPLE WITH MENTAL ILLNESS AND SEVERE LEARNING DISABILITIES

NHS Estates publications

HBN 35: Accommodation for people with mental illness:

Part 1 – The acute unit, HMSO, 1996.

Part 2 – Treatment with care in the community, HMSO, 1998.

Design Guide: Accommodation for adults with acute mental illness, HMSO, 1993.

Design Guide: Medium secure psychiatric units, HMSO, 1993.

Design Guide: Day facilities for people with severe learning disabilities, HMSO, 1993.

ACCOMMODATION FOR AMBULANCE SERVICES

NHS Estates publications

HBN 44: Accommodation for ambulance services, HMSO, 1994.

Other publications

Infection Control Nurses Association (2001), **Infection control practices for ambulance services**
http://www.icna.co.uk

About NHS Estates guidance and publications

The Agency has a dynamic fund of knowledge which it has acquired over 40 years of working in the field. Our unique access to estates and facilities data, policy and information is shared in guidance delivered in four principal areas:

Design & Building

These documents look at the issues involved in planning, briefing and designing facilities that reflect the latest developments and policy around service delivery. They provide current thinking on the best use of space, design and functionality for specific clinical services or non-clinical activity areas. They may contain schedules of accommodation. Guidance published under the headings Health Building Notes (HBNs) and Design Guides are found in this category.

Examples include:

HBN 54, Facilities for cancer care centres
HBN 28, Facilities for cardiac services
Diagnostic and Treatment Centres: ACAD, Central Middlesex Hospital – an evaluation
Infection control in the built environment: design and planning

Engineering & Operational (including Facilities Management, Fire, Health & Safety and Environment)

These documents provide guidance on the design, installation and running of specialised building service systems and also policy guidance and instruction on Fire, Health & Safety and Environment issues. Health Technical Memoranda (HTMs) and Health Guidance Notes (HGNs) are included in this category.

Examples include:

HTM 2007, Electrical services supply and distribution
HTM 2010, Sterilization: operational management with testing and validation protocols
HTM 2040, The control of legionellae in healthcare premises – a code of practice
HTM 82, Fire safety – alarm and detection systems

Procurement & Property

These are documents which deal with areas of broad strategic concern and planning issues, including capital and procurement.

Examples of titles published under this heading are:

Estatecode
How to Cost a Hospital
Developing an Estate Strategy
Sustainable Development in the NHS

NHS Estates Policy Initiatives

In response to some of the key tasks of the NHS Plan and the Modernisation Agenda, NHS Estates has implemented, project-managed and monitored several programmes for reform to improve the overall patient experience. These publications document the project outcomes and share best practice and data with the field.

Examples include:

National standards of cleanliness for the NHS
NHS Menu and Recipe Books
Sold on Health

The majority of publications are available in hard copy from:

The Stationery Office Ltd
PO Box 29, Norwich NR3 1GN
Telephone orders/General enquiries 0870 600 5522
Fax orders 0870 600 5533
E-mail book.orders@tso.co.uk
http://www.tso.co.uk/bookshop

Publication lists and selected downloadable publications can be found on our website:
http://www.nhsestates.gov.uk

For further information please contact our Information Centre:
e-mail: nhs.estates@doh.gsi.gov.uk
tel: 0113 254 7070